# TOOLS

## for the

# TOP PADDOCK

**Kane Brisco** is a Taranaki dairy farmer, public speaker, personal trainer, and father of three. After a successful farming career, he established FarmFit in 2019 as a functional fitness class for his local community, and it has since expanded into an online community of over 15,000 followers who subscribe to Kane's tips and advice on mental and physical wellbeing. This is his first book.

**Steve Kilgallon** is a national correspondent for *Stuff* and the *Sunday Star-Times*, specialising in investigative journalism and long-form feature writing. A lifelong city dweller, he has learned a lot about farming from the writing of this book, his fourth, after *The Sports Insider*, with athletics coach Jack Ralston; *Never Give Up*, with gas-explosion survivor Ian Winson; and *Relentless*, with Scott Donaldson, the first person to kayak the Tasman solo. Steve lives in Auckland with his partner and three children.

# TOOLS

## for the

# TOP PADDOCK

KANE BRISCO

with Steve Kilgallon

HarperCollins*Publishers*

**IMPORTANT INFORMATION**
This book provides general information regarding health, wellness, and physical exercise but does not take account of individual circumstances and this book is not in any way a substitute for medical advice or counselling. Before starting any new exercise, diet or weight-loss program, please consult with a qualified medical practitioner, qualified personal trainer and nutritionist or dietitian to ensure the recommendations meet your specific needs, especially if you have a pre-existing medical condition. The author and publisher do not accept any liability for any injury, loss, or damage that may arise from reliance on the information contained in this book.

**HarperCollins*Publishers***
Australia • Brazil • Canada • France • Germany • Holland • India
Italy • Japan • Mexico • New Zealand • Poland • Spain • Sweden
Switzerland • United Kingdom • United States of America

First published in 2022
by HarperCollins*Publishers* (New Zealand) Limited
Unit D1, 63 Apollo Drive, Rosedale, Auckland 0632, New Zealand
harpercollins.co.nz



A catalogue record for this book is available from the National Library of New Zealand

ISBN 978 1 7755 4212 4 (pbk)
ISBN 978 1 7754 9243 6 (ebook)

Cover design by Christine Armstrong, HarperCollins Design Studio
Cover image by Lottie Hedley
Typeset in Sabon LT Std by Kirby Jones
Printed and bound in Australia by McPherson's Printing Group

If this book raises any concerns for you or someone you love, you can access help at any of the below organisations:

Lifeline 0800 543 354 (0800 LIFELINE)

Suicide Crisis Helpline 0508 828 865 (0508 TAUTOKO)

Depression and Anxiety Helpline 0800 111 757

Are You OK (family violence helpline) 0800 456 450

Rape Crisis 0800 883 300

Rural Support 0800 787 254

Need to Talk – Text or call 1737

Will to Live – www.willtolivenz.com

I Am Hope – www.iamhope.org.nz

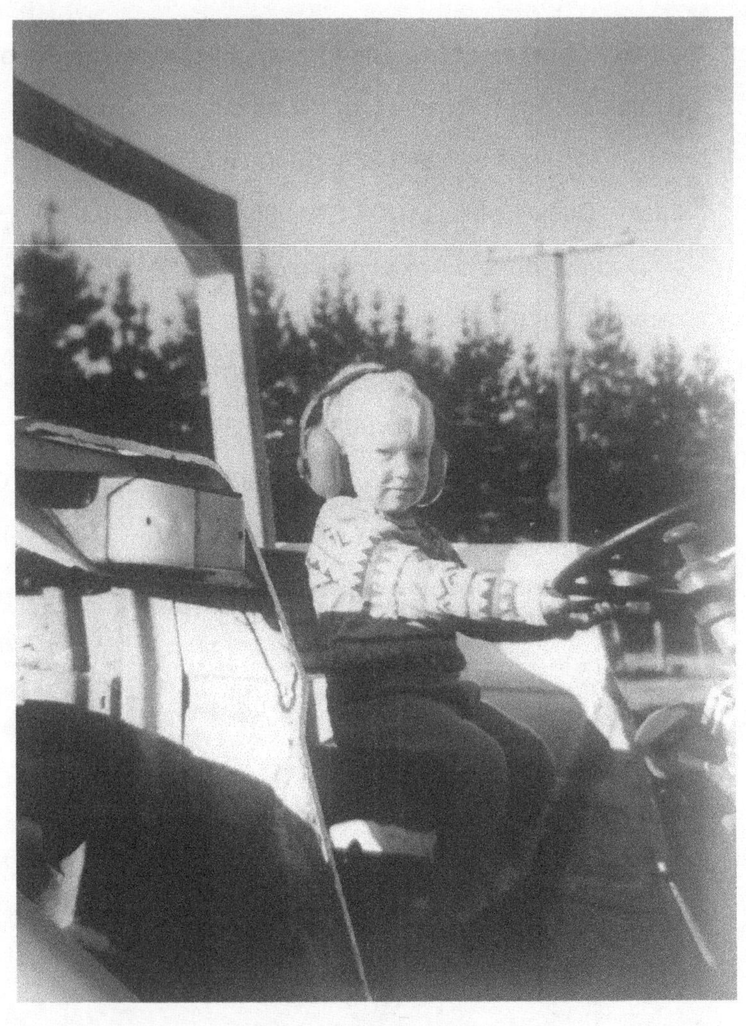

*As a four-year old on my favourite farm vehicle,*
*Uncle Ian's Ford Tractor.*

# Contents

Introduction 1

1: Turning Pain into Positives 7
2: Growing Resilience 21
3: Learning to Breathe 49
4: 'Who' is More Important than 'Where' 81
5: Mental Health Needs Physical Support 99
6: Home Truths 127
7: Going Back to Go Forwards 147
8: Keeping Original 169
9: FarmFit at Home 193
10: The Circle of Life 211
11: Adapting and Overcoming 225
12: Embracing Uncertainty 251

Acknowledgements 279

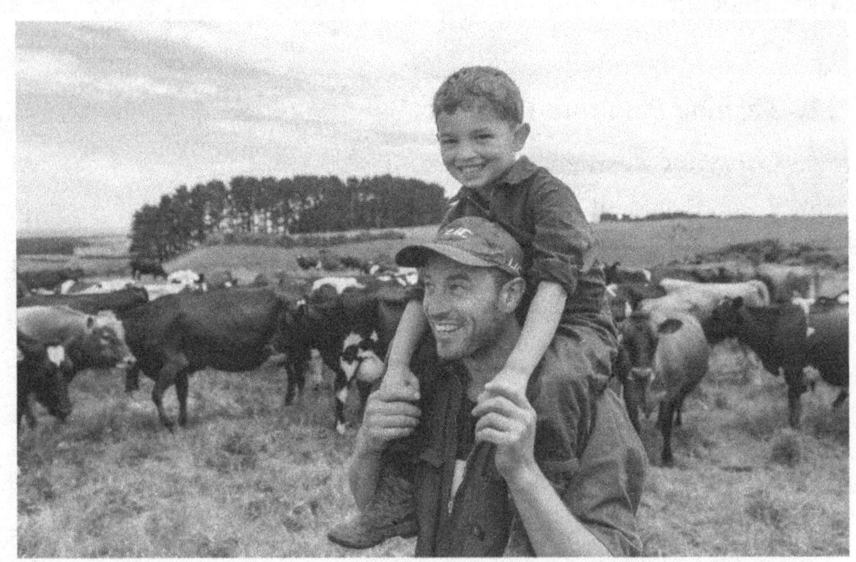

*Me and my right-hand-man, Parker, checking the cows.*

# Introduction

FIVE YEARS AGO, if I'd seen myself holding up my phone and talking into it, I'd have given myself a punch in the guts and reminded myself that such stuff was for the show-offs up in town. That's not what a Kiwi farmer does, and I was that farmer: a typical, stoic, hide-your-emotions stereotype who didn't like being photographed or even noticed. Now I've got social media accounts with over 13,000 followers, where I talk openly about mental and physical fitness.

The Instagram account emerged out of FarmFit, a bootcamp-style functional fitness programme run for the local community from my Taranaki farm.

And FarmFit had its genesis in a very dark place. A year earlier, life was bleak for me. A tough few years on the farm, with droughts and record low prices for the milk we produced, left me in a deep financial hole, compounded to leave me questioning whether I still wanted to be a farmer, and whether, indeed, I was any good at farming. Digging myself out of that low was the catalyst for a huge change in my mindset.

I was one of those people who would go on to Facebook – not to share something of my life, but to get stuck into an argument with some stranger I disagreed with. I don't know why I did it – perhaps to distract myself from the real issues in life I wasn't yet ready to deal with.

But I soon realised that nobody wins from arguing online – it's bloody stupid, and I had to remind myself I'd been brought up to understand that if you can't say it to someone's face, it's best not to say it at all.

My other realisation was that most of the people on social media were complaining about life, almost waiting for someone to come and help them, and to fix their problems for them. Mental health had become a hot topic – especially in the rural sector, where there had been a spate of suicides – and a lot of people were blaming the government for not funding enough services. As an aside, I believe that's true: there's an ambulance waiting at the bottom of the cliff but nothing to provide a safety net for those at the top of the cliff. I also believe it's up to you to start building your own safety net to stop yourself falling off that cliff, to start taking some personal responsibility. I constructed my net through a journey of discovery, learning about myself and from the wins and losses of life. I wanted to get that message out there – that the ultimate responsibility for our mental health lies with us, and we shouldn't wait for someone else to do it for us.

FarmFit was another way to continue challenging myself, mentally and physically. My approach has always been to stretch myself and attempt things that make me feel uncomfortable. I'd always hated being on camera and you won't find many photographs of me. It took me outside my comfort zone. I realised that – not only to be successful and to farm into a changing future, but also to be successful in life – we need to adapt, understand and grow. Growth needs an open mind. That's how you give yourself a lot more options and opportunities in all aspects of life. A closed mindset will never open any doors.

My videos are real. They are honest and they are direct. They also contain a fair bit of swearing. I've only got one approach. I say what I think, and deal with the consequences afterwards and, while that has caused me some issues, I wouldn't change it, because we could all do with some brutal honesty from time to time. I particularly wanted to challenge the archetype of the stoic Kiwi rural male, and the drawbacks attached to that failure to show your emotions.

My messages have never been about what I have been through personally, more about the lessons that I have learned along the way. I never wanted sympathy or empathy. Most of the stories in this book I've never shared before, but the ups and downs I've traversed do explain what I have learned.

Every chapter in my life has provided me with a major lesson, and along the journey I've also picked up some tips, quotes and mindsets that have helped me just as much.

Hopefully I've been just as honest as I am online.

Actually, the tipping point in my decision to write this book was when I told my two brothers about the idea. They both laughed at me and said, 'No, I wouldn't buy it.' And I said, 'Well, I'm definitely doing it then.' They provided me with plenty of motivation to write this book. I also hope they are wrong, and that anyone – farmer or not – can find something in it that will make them think, challenge their mindset, and help them with whatever troubles they might face.

**Kane Brisco, January 2022**

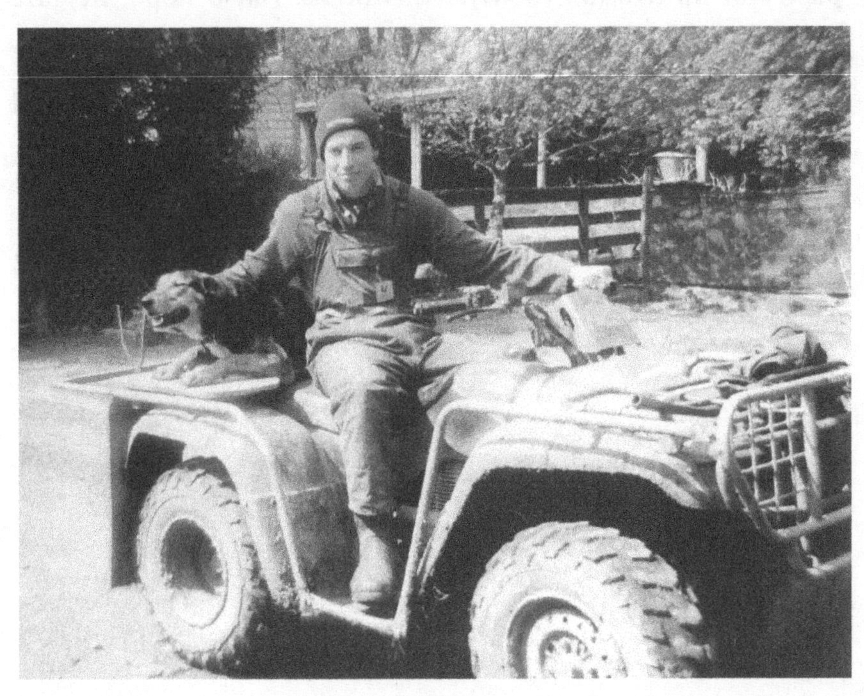

*As a fresh-faced 19-year-old stockman,*
*with my first dog, King.*

# Chapter one

# Turning Pain into Positives

I COULD MILK A COW by the time I turned five. When Uncle Ian's alarm went off at 4am, I would be up, dressed in my overalls, and ready to go to work on the farm. For as long as I could remember, I wanted to be a farmer. The only problem was, I didn't live on a farm – I was only a visitor.

Instead, I was born in Waitara, a small freezing works and petrochemical town with a bit of a reputation close to New Plymouth, in Taranaki, on the west coast of New Zealand's North Island. My dad, Ian, was a mechanic and my mother, Glenys, raised her three sons, but always worked part- or full-time in all sorts of jobs from cleaning to catering. They were very hardworking, honest and selfless, and I think it's testament to them that – despite my two brothers and I travelling some rocky roads and having our troubles – I think we've turned into good humans who retain the values they instilled in us.

But being a townie by birth didn't stop me being a farmer in spirit. I can blame that on my uncle, Ian McCaul, who had the family dairy farm, Kowhai Ayrshire Stud, not far from

Waitara, which he had taken over at the age of 16 when his father died.

I have two much older brothers – half-brothers, technically, as their father had passed away many years earlier. Nathan is 11 years older than me, and Miah nine, and I spent a lot of my early life trying to keep up with them.

The three of us would be shipped out to Uncle Ian's farm on weekends and holidays, and that's where we all fell in love with farming. Once that early morning alarm went off, I would be his shadow for the day, whether he liked it or not. My brothers had been just the same before me, and Nathan and Miah would both go on to become dairy farmers. They also each left home when they were 16, so I had much of my childhood as an only child.

Like most kids I knew, I loved being outside kicking a ball, riding my bike, building stuff, or – my favourite – taking things apart to see how they worked; but most of all, I loved being out on the farm.

Uncle Ian is your real typical old-school Kiwi bloke; he wore an old check shirt, black rugby shorts, overalls with the sleeves hacked off and Red Band gumboots every day of the week, every week of the year. He worked every day of his life, and built everything himself, even his own boat.

I can vividly remember late nights falling asleep on an old couch out in the shed while Uncle Ian and his mate Murray Nicholls toiled away on what seemed to be a never-ending DIY project, with the smell of Black Heart rum, Port Royal smokes, and sawdust combining to send me off to sleep. At the time, Uncle Ian had no kids of his own, but he was the cool uncle, something like an extra dad.

Uncle Ian had a pedigree Ayrshire herd and used to show his cows at country shows, so we learned stockmanship and what a good cow looked like pretty early on.

Unusually, my Nana also lived in the same house. It was the same one she had moved into when she was married in 1948, at the age of 22. My brothers and I spent a great deal of our childhood listening to, and – most importantly – watching someone who'd been born between the wars and had worked a farm fulltime since she was 13.

I say watched for a reason. Nana didn't talk much – she just did whatever needed doing, whenever it needed to be done, without complaint. My generation could, and did, learn a lot from her.

To this day, Nana McCaul is the toughest person I know, and someone we all look up to.

**Don't spend so much time thinking, talking, and moaning about doing. Be like Nana McCaul, and just f**king do it.**

Spending time with Uncle Ian and Nana McCaul gave us a taste of the typical farm upbringing: riding quad bikes, driving tractors, and being free to roam and explore from a very young age. We were allowed to find our own mischief, but Uncle Ian often led the way in pushing those boundaries: a favourite trick was trying to tip us kids out of the tractor bucket as we drove around the farm. You wouldn't get away with a lot of it these days.

When my mum picked me up from the farm on a Sunday evening, I'd hide from her to try and avoid going home. At school, I used to just daydream about being back on the farm.

When I was about five, we moved to Bell Block, a nice little town just outside New Plymouth, the largest city in Taranaki, I assume to be near the high school where my brothers attended.

It was a good upbringing and a great place to grow up. Throughout, Mum and Dad gave me some free reign to make my own decisions and, most importantly, take responsibility for my own actions.

I reckon I had a great relationship with my parents, but over time, things did become a little strained with my dad. I think I acquired a lot of my characteristics from him: he was a perfectionist and, I think, quite highly strung. He always gave 100 per cent to his work and, like me, was something of a workaholic. It meant we didn't always see much of him and, at times, I felt as if he didn't have a lot of time for me.

Not until I became a dad myself did I really understand that, and that I had started doing the same thing with my kids. I understood then the natural responsibility a parent feels to provide an easier life for their family, and that sometimes prioritising them means being away from them.

I didn't appreciate it at the time, but now I know that he showed me sacrifice and hard work are a requirement for success.

When I was young, I had a pretty bad year; a year that had a huge impact on the rest of my life.

A boy who was several years older than me sexually abused me over the course of about six months. It was very confusing. I knew it was wrong. But I wasn't old enough to fully understand it and it wasn't until some years later that I really started processing it and understanding what had happened to me.

The abuse began with persuasion, then quickly turned to threats. He was much bigger and stronger and, at that age, I didn't understand what was happening. Any hesitation or refusal was met with threats, so I became compliant. For a long time, I hated myself for not being stronger, for not telling someone, or doing more to stop it. I blamed myself. I can remember wanting to tell someone, but I also remember that feeling of shame – that it was my fault for allowing it to happen, and I would be judged harshly if anybody knew. I felt helpless and, ultimately, that I had let myself down.

I'm revealing this part of my life not just because of the impact it had on me, but also because male sexual abuse is so rarely talked about, and it is much more common than I ever thought it would be. It's hard to find exact numbers, but about one in four women, and about one in ten men suffer some type of sexual abuse. But throughout most of my life it felt like it must be closer to one in a million – and I was that unlucky bastard.

It was around the same time that I also overheard my uncle, whom I worshipped, talking to one of his mates about me in a rather unflattering way: along the lines that I was 'not the sharpest tool in the shed'. It was heartbreaking to hear my hero say, in effect, that I wasn't going to amount to much.

It confirmed something I already believed: a good farmer needed common sense and a smart mind, and I possessed neither. I never felt as if I had that clichéd Number 8 wire ability.

Hearing my worst beliefs about my own character confirmed stripped me of some of that deep love of farming.

I was already a very shy boy. My brothers are both quite loud and confident, but I was a quiet, bashful little fellow. And whatever confidence I might have possessed was shattered by these two pivotal events.

I think a consequence of any physical or sexual abuse leaves the survivor constantly assessing potential threats. I became a people watcher, always evaluating everyone I met to see if they posed any threat to me. As I became older, I developed a sense of people's energy, their words and actions, and why they said and did what they did. I'm sure many people do, but mine felt heightened and refined by the abuse I had endured.

I really retreated from life, and, going into my teenage years, I remained a very self-conscious, quiet boy who lacked confidence.

But I also had a deep-seated anger; a hatred of what had happened to me. I didn't let it out often, but I knew it was there. When it did come out, it was directed at other people, or at the world.

## Anger that isn't dealt with turns to hate.

Pivotal moments in our journey through life define our characters. Hopefully, these are mostly positive experiences. Unfortunately for me, two of my most significant moments were anything but. These two experiences shaped my otherwise-typical childhood and combined to dent my confidence – and that feeling of helplessness held me back for many years to come.

Trying to turn those experiences into positives was my way out. I think the first time I managed to turn that pain into a positive was on the rugby field. I played fullback, and we had just begun playing the full-contact version of the game. I was not a confrontational player; I'd run around defenders, never at them. In one game against our local rivals, someone kicked me in the guts in a ruck. I was too scared to retaliate, but I felt the anger grow until I was enraged. I received the ball downfield and carried it at full tilt into the first defender I spotted; I can even recall letting out something like a war cry as we collided.

To my surprise I bowled him over, and kept charging upfield. I remember seeing the surprise on my teammates' faces, and I suspect it would have looked pretty funny to everyone else. I had these rare moments of bravery growing up, but I couldn't understand where they came from, or how to control it. I didn't know it then, but with time I would learn.

Much later in life, I came to realise that I probably spent a lot of time reacting to those two significant events: proving to my abuser and to my uncle that they were wrong.

Reading about the abuse will come as a surprise to many people who know me. I never told anyone about it until years later and, until now, only a few people knew about it.

It took a lot away from me, but it's given me a lot more than it has taken. I doubt you would hear many people say that about their abuse. That's been my choice, and I used that pain as a positive – as a motivating tool to perform well in rugby, boxing, and farming. I sought out and found the positives in a negative experience. A lot of people don't find that outlet, and it's a huge weight to carry without being able to express it – or expressing it negatively, in substance abuse, depression, or abusing others.

**Pressure bursts pipes. Holding onto trauma like this – no matter how far down you shove it – always builds pressure over time. I feel so lucky that I discovered a way to release that pressure in a safe and positive manner.**

When I took up boxing, to be honest, one reason was probably so that one day I could go and give him a hiding. The other option was to press charges. I've never really considered doing that. It's tough though, because I would be absolutely mortified if I found out that he did the same to someone else later on in life; and yet, on the other hand, he might have a family now. Do I rip all that down all these years later? I don't know if anyone would be a winner if he were to be charged and went to court. So I dealt with it in my own way, and continue to deal with it in a positive way. To me that's enough – I can live with it – but I wish I had told someone at the time and asked for help.

I think much of my life was a journey of hiding that secret, burying it deep down inside to try and forget it, and almost erasing it – while not realising its enduring impact on me. Having your boundaries broken creates a lot of feelings, mostly anger and resentment. It was years later that I understood I had to face up to it – then let go of it – and the only way to achieve that was finding forgiveness.

I struggled with that concept for a long time. How can you forgive someone for doing something so horrible? You don't! I had to forgive myself. It wasn't the abuse that was hurting me, but holding onto it still gave him power over me. Why should I let that small time in my life taint the rest of it? No. I had to forgive my younger self, and accept that I'd done the best I could at the time.

## You can't judge the past with the knowledge you have now.

Likewise, I have never ever spoken to my uncle about what I had overheard him say. And I should make it clear he became a very big supporter of me. I doubt he would even remember saying it. I've even run through the conversation in my head where I confront him about it, and I can just imagine him saying: 'I wouldn't have said that.' It was just an off-the-cuff thing he said to his mate, but, as a young boy, it broke my heart.

It was another source of pain that I turned into motivation, and it was an experience that helped me set definite goals around my farming career.

So, as much as those two incidents hurt me deeply when they happened, and caused me some ongoing pain, I know I wouldn't have made it to where I am now without them.

I love it when people doubt me, it's fuel on the fire for me, so I just have to prove them wrong; just like my brothers saying they wouldn't read this book. You're already a chapter in, lads! Sometimes you need someone to doubt you.

TOP PADDOCK TOOL

## Turning Pain into a Positive

I don't know that this is advice that any psychologist or counsellor would dispense. I'm sure some of them would specifically advise against it if it meant you never sought the proper support – and they'd be right about that.

But the reality is that it takes a lot of strength and a lot of time to be able to really work through your trauma, to talk about it and learn to heal. In the interim, people are going to turn that pain into something, and finding a positive outlet for it may be the healthiest way to deal with it.

I know that in my teenage years, I certainly buried my abuse as deep as it could possibly go. It was when I took up boxing that I began to understand that I could turn my pain into a positive, and I could actually take something from the experience. I've used the abuse – and, to a lesser extent, that comment by my uncle – as a motivational force. Now when I speak in public, I talk about turning pain into a positive, because I have used those key moments as motivation to do well.

A deeply traumatic experience does not have to ruin the rest of your life. I certainly haven't allowed mine to. I discovered I could choose to control it, and turn it into a positive.

I must stress that this isn't therapy, and this isn't a substitute for it. But some people, myself included, take many years before they are able to talk to anyone about their trauma, and this was the only way I found to release some of that pain. It was a way of getting on with life, until I was strong enough to properly work through it. Ideally, you'd use this advice and have therapy as well.

It worked for me for nearly 20 years, allowing me to have a positive outlook on life, rather than heading down the path of alcohol and drug abuse that unfortunately so many people take when they cannot find such a positive outlet.

In a rudimentary way, I was working my way through the pain because pushing myself to the limits – and to a point that most people never reach – does make you face your demons. For example, in boxing I'd reach a point where I was so exhausted that even lifting my arms into a defensive guard felt like too much. At that point, I would picture my abuser's face on my opponent's body, and that would allow me to get past that fatigue barrier and keep fighting. The anger turned into fuel. When I used that technique repeatedly, I understood that I could control it, and it no longer controlled me. In the ring, when you get angry, you get sloppy, and you get hit. I was able to use it in a controlled manner to keep going, and I've since used it in farming, and in running when I've reached points where I felt I couldn't keep going. Training and competing requires a level of pain and suffering, but that suffering in no way compares to the suffering of a traumatic experience. When I was doing hill running, and the lactic acid filled my legs, and my lungs began to burn, I would say to myself, 'This is not as painful as that was.' The worst experience you've ever been through in your life can be used as fuel to turn your mindset around.

In my early twenties, I felt I had come to terms with the abuse and was able to forgive myself. It was a big step and, later on, when I began FarmFit, I realised that if the abuse had never happened I may not have been spurred on to achieve in life. In that way, it became a horrible gift.

The bad things that happen in life are often the making of you. I wouldn't wish what happened to me on anyone – but I've used it to make me who I am today, and that's one of my best achievements. The tough experiences that give us the challenges in life can drive us to produce something extra in ourselves.

It's not the victories, achievements and celebrations that really determine who we are. It's the challenges, struggles and defeats – and the way we respond to them – that define our character. Make yours a positive definition.

## Chapter two

# Growing Resilience

I PLAYED RUGBY FROM around the age of five. It was inevitable; both my brothers played rugby, and I looked up to them. But I was just an average player. I didn't make any representative teams. Throughout childhood and my teen years, I tried a host of sports – I really enjoyed cricket, squash, indoor soccer and athletics – and while I always picked up the skills quickly, absolute bang average was as far as I got with any of them.

The only trophy I ever won was one I got at the age of eight, for being the most dedicated. It didn't stop me dreaming of being an All Black though; rugby and farming were my only real dreams, and I was absolutely mad on both of them.

I kept playing through high school, and in my final year at New Plymouth Boys High, I played for the Fifth XV. If you were wondering, that was the worst XV the school fielded.

I really enjoyed sport. It never bothered me that I never made trials or rep teams. I was just happy to be out on the field getting amongst it. I think everything we get out of sport is in the journey; the longer you stick at it the more you learn.

**Winners aren't necessarily happy just about the win, they're happy about everything they overcame, the discipline and hard work they went through. If you're not learning and growing, then you're not really winning.**

I decided that year I was going to leave school. I reached an agreement with my parents that if I saw out the year, they would help me buy my first car. But I didn't put a lot of effort in. A fair bit of that final year was spent at the beach trying to surf, or at friends' places playing guitar or listening to music. I found music incredibly helpful in dealing with the confusion in my life at that time.

I didn't pass the year. I don't remember being particularly worried about that. Then Dad said: 'Well, if you're not going to be at school you need to get a job.'

I had absolutely no idea what I really wanted to do. Dairy farming was the easy option, because I knew I could get a job. I still had an enduring love of farming, but at that age, the thought of rising before 5am seven days a week wasn't particularly appealing. My parents, however, had no intention of allowing me to stay under their roof and sit on my arse. I was shipped off to live with my oldest brother, Nathan, who had kindly offered to take me off their hands.

Nathan was living about 90 minutes' drive south, just outside the small town of Patea, where he was share-milking a herd of 400 cows. So, as a runty little 17-year-old, I found myself living in a sleepout in Nathan's garage, milking his cows to pay the rent, and picking up relief milking work (going to milk other farmers' cows when they needed a day off) to earn a bit of cash. Nathan suggested that, since I was living there, I should join him at the local rugby club, Border. At first I politely declined, because I weighed about 65kg and I had watched the giants he played against. I was average enough playing against people my own size, let alone anyone twice as big.

But my brother weighed about 120kg, and had bright red hair and a matching temper. Not many people say no to Old Red – he simply said: 'Ah, no, you're coming.' I saw out the remainder of that season sitting on the bench, not getting much game time. When I did get on the field, I was pretty bloody average.

But in the off-season, the rugby club decided to organise a boxing tournament as a fundraiser.

It was around the time that corporate boxing was beginning to take off, thanks to the televised Fight for Life series promoted by former Kiwi rugby league international Dean Lonergan, which pitched retired sportspeople and celebrities into the ring.

I'm not sure why I volunteered – it was entirely out of character. I was not a confrontational person, and I hadn't been in many fights at school. But as a kid I'd idolised Mike Tyson.

Tyson had been in his prime around the time I was abused. And I think I wanted to be like him because I felt that, if I was a bad b*stard like Tyson, nobody would touch me the way that kid had. In reality, I was the opposite: small, weak and I couldn't defend myself, but I didn't much like that state of affairs.

Eight or nine of us from the rugby club signed up, and an old guy from Patea named Dennis McKenna, a former New Zealand champion who was about 70 years old, came along a couple of times a week to train us. And I absolutely fell in love with boxing.

I'd never really trained properly before. It was all new, I was learning some skills and I found I picked it up quite well – probably better than most of the other guys. I discovered boxing was a great leveller: it doesn't matter if you're rich or poor, how big you are, or the logo on your shirt. Boxing is about character, discipline, smarts, the ability to be calm in chaos, and to get even, not angry.

The fight was held in February. Also on the bill was my brother Red, one of the fight organisers. His opponent withdrew three weeks before fight night, so my other brother Miah put his hand up. Because he hadn't had time to get his registration and medical clearance, they called it an exhibition fight, which meant no scores could be registered and the bout was automatically considered a draw. To this day, there's much debate as to who really won. It was quite a heated bout. Mum had her eyes closed the whole time, and was in tears by the end.

When it came to my fight, I knew the guy I was matched against, and I was pretty confident I was going to win. I was scheduled for the first fight of the night. I'll never forget that moment: I've never been so bloody nervous in my life. It was a horrible feeling. When the bell rang, you could have heard a pin drop. It was terrifying.

The adrenaline rushed into my body, the energy drained away, and it felt like my hands were holding concrete bricks. Panic set in, and I can tell you that's a horrible feeling to experience 30 seconds into round one, when you know there's still a long way to go. It was a vastly different experience to the sparring I'd done in training, and I distinctly remember how my senses were heightened, and tunnel vision set in.

**No matter how well prepared you are, if you can't control your nervous system when it comes time to perform, then all of that preparation is forgotten. Be in the moment, not in the future. Without the ability to focus on what's right in front of you, a lot of what you know goes out of your head.**

I was fitter than I'd ever been, and confident in my boxing abilities. Despite all those nerves I put up a pretty good display, and won with a fair margin.

Those six minutes of boxing were the most uncomfortable, challenging six minutes I had ever been a willing participant in; but they were also the most exhilarating, exciting, and life changing. The only way I can describe it is to say that I walked into that ring as one person, and walked out another.

**Boxing taught me to be calm in the chaos. When you're calm, you can see everything clearly; your mind remains in your logical-thinking, well-developed frontal lobe. When this part of the brain is in control, it's much easier to react well and keep your energy focused in the right place.**

I left with a massive sense of accomplishment and a huge boost to my general confidence, because I had achieved something I never thought I would. I had never imagined I would be courageous enough to step into a boxing ring, I hadn't thought it was something I had in me. But somehow part of me had driven me to do it and, in the process, told that doubting voice in my mind to piss off. I had proven it wrong and, in turn, proven something to myself.

I believe that was a significant turning point in my life. It began to rebuild the confidence I had lost as a scared young boy, and it changed my mindset. As a teenager, I didn't do exciting things. I didn't test myself or take risks because I didn't want to experience discomfort.

I kept up the boxing. For six months, I trained in Whanganui, but never got a fight down there. Then I found a trainer in Normanby, about a 40 minute drive inland. Steve Hartley, who is now the president of Boxing New Zealand, had a great reputation as a boxing coach, and it was fortunate for me that he took me under his wing. Over the next few years, I had another five amateur fights as one of his boxers.

My time training with Steve began to show what boxing could offer me in other areas of my life: transferable skills such as calmness, discipline, intelligence under pressure, skills that I'd lacked when growing up. I was now practising them almost every day and, if I could do it in the boxing ring, was there anything stopping me from doing it in other parts of my life?

It seeded another dream: I felt such an immediate impact from boxing, and a love of it, that I wanted to pass on not just the skills but also the life lessons I derived from it.

**In many ways, life itself is just like a fight.**

I learned another key lesson when Steve took me to Palmerston North for my second fight. I remember going to the weigh-in, and Steve pointed out the guy I was matched against. He just looked like a typical white guy, nothing to be worried about.

He had a tracksuit on, zipped to the neck, but when he went to the scales, he took the tracksuit off, and he was covered head to toe in tattoos. 'F**king hell,' I thought, 'I've got no tattoos.' All of a sudden he looked mean and tough. I turned to Steve with a look that said, 'What have you done here? Is this a set-up?' I was still battling my self-confidence at this point. Steve just said: 'Tough stickers don't make you tough.' Then he said something else that was quite an important lesson for me too, something along the lines of that he had put me in there because of my ability, and he believed I was better than the other guy. 'Just do what you've trained to do,' he said. 'Don't worry about the outcome: that will take care of itself if you just do what you've done in training.'

**Confidence comes from competence. Sometimes we need a reminder that we've done the hard work. You'll never truly have confidence if you know you haven't done all you need to. Cutting corners always has a price.**

As soon as I'd seen the tattoos, I'd assumed the other guy was a hard man, and he was going to smash me. But that little bit of reassurance, the reminder that I'd done the training, that I was technically sound and capable, and to trust in what I had learned, kept me calm.

It was a tougher fight than my first. But, as Steve had told me, I had the ability, and I was able to think, listen, and act under pressure. Another win, and I was presented with my first trophy in nearly 20 years.

That fight consolidated some lessons I was learning about life. I was learning to do what I'd previously thought impossible. I was learning to rely on myself, that I didn't need Mum and Dad to hold my hand, and I didn't need a team alongside me or a training partner to motivate me.

**Vulnerability is the state that sets combat sports apart. Everything about you is on show to the audience: your willpower, the way you handle adversity, whether you've trained hard enough, or cut corners. There's nowhere to hide in the ring and no one to help. The truth comes out, whether you like it or not.**

Another positive consequence of my new-found love of boxing was that it transformed my rugby. The next season, I went from being on the bench to the starting side. And by halfway through the season, I was playing a full game for the club's second team, then jumping on the bench for the senior team, relishing every chance I got to play some minutes for them.

The following season, I was a starting player in the first team, and even made the Taranaki under-20s representative team. That meant a lot to me: I had always been a big Taranaki supporter, so to wear the amber and black colours made me incredibly proud, all the more so because I felt someone like me was never, ever meant to. I was shocked to even be invited to trial in the first place.

That first season of senior rugby I weighed just over 70kg, and played flanker, a position in the forwards normally taken by blokes weighing 100kg or more.

I would go on to play about 130 senior games for the Border rugby club.

I held my own. I took a lot of big knocks, but I got back up and kept going. It taught me about toughing things out, physically and mentally, and it made me stronger. Being smaller meant I had to go harder, and put more effort in. I think I began to gain more respect from people, particularly in the rugby environment.

**Don't let someone else's advantages become your disadvantage.**

**Never let your genetics or your past be an excuse for not achieving your goals. Yes, it makes it harder if you're not naturally blessed, but it also offers the opportunity to go to places – mentally and physically – that the gifted don't travel to. It adds character, and that gives you something extra. It's only a weakness if you want to be.**

Some of the bigger blokes would try to take advantage of my size on the field, and there were times when I would end up in fights with the biggest member of the other team, but I would never back down.

Not long into that season we were up against Southern, in our local derby match. I was our starting flanker, up against a pack containing several Taranaki rep players. From the very first scrum, the opposing flanker began holding my jersey, preventing me from taking off from the scrum to make the first tackle. I told one of my teammates what was happening. He said: 'What are you telling me for? Do something about it.'

I wasn't quite sure what he meant. We got to the next scrum, and the opposing player did it again. I whacked his arm away and told him to cut it out. He laughed his head off and asked what I was going to do about it, and grabbed my collar again.

Next scrum he did it again, again I shoved him away, but this time, the scrum was already finishing up and I was beginning to stand up when he grabbed me again. 'Perfect,' I thought.

I ducked down, so he ended up grabbing my jersey more on the back of my shoulder – which was exactly what I wanted. Boxing had taught me a lot about transferring strength from the ground to my fists, and the mechanics behind generating power. His right hand was holding my jersey, and I was crouched lower than him with my left foot close to his body.

That let me line up his liver, ripe for me to unleash a short left hook. He yelped like a dog and hunched over. His teammates looked confused, mine laughed, and sledged him. He looked embarrassed, and was really confused about what had happened. I ended up with a major confidence boost and a feeling of empowerment.

**Feeling safe can be the result of being strong. I had often sought out security, comfort, and shelter to keep me safe. I realised that out on that rugby field, my boxing skills and new-found strength and fitness provided me with more safety than I thought possible: 'Better to be a warrior in a garden than a gardener in a war.'**

I was extremely proud of making the Taranaki under-20s team and wearing the province's amber and black colours. Shane McDonald, who played nine years and 116 games for the province, and Andy Slater, who played 13 years and 180 games, were the coaches. I could remember running on to the field at Yarrow Stadium as a kid, getting their autographs when Taranaki beat North Harbour to defend the Ranfurly Shield in 1996.

After the pre-season games I went to see Steve to tell him I didn't think I could still box, train, and play rugby in New

Plymouth: something had to give. He said: 'If you've got half a chance at making money at rugby, go and do that, because it's a lot easier than boxing.'

I wasn't in the Taranaki starting side, but I played about half of the season's eight games. Our first pre-season game was against a very physically developed Waikato team who all looked about three years older than us. They were well-drilled and hammered us, but I got on for the final 20 minutes, went bloody hard, and played a blinder, forcing a couple of turnovers and a penalty, and making some good tackles. It earned me a start the following week against Whanganui.

Around this time, I fell ill and was unwell for about three months. I was working hard on the farm all day, dagging sheep, fencing, spraying weeds ... and being a young bloke living alone, I didn't know much about nutrition. I didn't know what a calorie was, how much I should eat, or how important protein was to developing strength and repairing muscle. I was training six nights a week, and didn't realise I wasn't eating what I needed to in order to support that workload.

**Stress is stress. The body doesn't differentiate between different types – training, work, physical, or emotional – it all just compounds, and that illness was the result. It sucked.**

At the end of that season, Andy sat me down and said I had all the attributes to be a good rugby player: I was determined, smart, a good communicator, and a leader, but I needed to put on 25kg to be competitive at the next level.

So a month after the season ended, I walked into a gym, weighing around 71kg. I told the owner my situation, bought a three-month membership, and I went there religiously every second night and lifted weights. I bought a big bag of protein powder, went on a body-building programme, and walked out of that gym a few months later weighing 87kg.

Andy reckoned I needed to be at 95–100kg, but I thought 87kg was pretty good, and I could go through the season at that weight, then bulk up some more in the next off-season.

**Just because you're not a professional, doesn't mean you can't behave like one. Your attitude towards something, and the habits you create to support that, cost nothing.**

I soon learned that a body-building program didn't work on the rugby field. I couldn't run like I used to, and I felt terribly unfit. I didn't have a very good season, but it was a good learning experience. It was the first time I'd set foot in a gym and, to be honest, I haven't really been into one since. But it was good that I could take the discipline I'd gained from boxing and apply it into a different physical pursuit.

I attributed my huge improvement in rugby to what I had learned from boxing. I was no longer scared of anyone on the field. In fact, I wasn't intimidated by anyone. I could walk into a room and not feel afraid of other men. It was quite a powerful feeling, having spent my teenage years feeling intimidated by just about anyone. I didn't, at the time, understand it as well as I do now. I just went with it. But I did feel a change inside me. It was the start of a big journey for me – a journey I am still on.

I place a lot of value on taking skills from one area and using them in other areas of my life.

Boxing produced a complete change in how I saw life, and one area it had an impact in was rugby. It made me understand that going outside my comfort zone could give me something invaluable, and helped me learn and grow.

I learned much more about physical fitness from boxing than I ever did from rugby. In those days, you just did your own work. It was a small rural rugby club, and whatever state you turned up in for the first training session was what it was.

For example, boxing taught me how to breathe. When you start sparring, you actually forget to breathe: you're so tense you hold your breath. Then you learn that, when you punch, you should breathe out, and to remind yourself to do it, you make a huffing sound. Listen to boxers in a gym, and you can hear them all making that noise as they exhale. When your lungs are empty, your mind automatically knows how to refill them in any circumstance – but they will hold onto air when faced with fight, flight or freeze situations.

In between rounds, you get a minute to recover. The first part of that is spent getting your breath under control and lowering your heart rate, so that you're in a better position to start the next round. I learned how to consciously control my breathing. I saw that it worked, and I figured I could probably apply it to rugby. At every break in a game, I would practise my breathing and lower my heart rate, and that felt really good and benefited my performance. I also noticed that I'd feel a bit calmer. In high pressure situations, if I was angry or frustrated I would consciously control my breathing. Then I noticed that the All Blacks and the Warriors had brought in a ritual where, after a try, they would huddle together and take three big deep breaths to calm down.

The next step was applying it to farming.

I had a new job. It was originally meant to be a short-term gig, working on a local drystock farm, providing pasture grazing for cattle being fattened up for meat, down the road from my brother's place. That was good news for me, because I wasn't enjoying waking up at 4.30am to go and milk cows. Show me a 17-year-old who does.

I got the job at Cawood Farms because the farm manager, who'd been there for a long time, was leaving, and the owner, Martyn Dickie, who was in his sixties, was looking for a young bloke to help out over summer while he found a replacement.

The manager was still serving out his notice, so my job was to learn the ropes off him, and pick asparagus on the farm's cropping block in the downtime.

I really loved that job but I was still learning the role of managing such a big place, and how to deal with all the unexpected challenges that go hand in hand with working with the land, animals and mother nature. It was stressful – I spent long hours learning on the job as a young man replacing an experienced older man. I found myself becoming anxious, and even started to have panic attacks. I used the breathing techniques to calm me down.

I distinctly remember the first time I applied it on the farm. It was during a 24-hour period in which the nearby town had a one-in-a-hundred-year rainfall.

I recall going outside in the middle of the storm to check the stock, and saw the river that ran beside the farm was rapidly rising, effortlessly sweeping away our 3km of boundary fences. I shifted any nearby stock away from the river and into secure paddocks on higher ground, and then found out the river had taken out our water supply, which crossed over the river from a neighbouring property. It would not be an easy fix. Then I came across a group of young bull calves. Three were down, unable to rise and looking worse for wear, so I had to go and get the tractor, lift them onto a trailer, and take them into the sheds to warm them up. I called the vet because they were suffering from hypothermia and pneumonia. It was probably my first big weather challenge in farming, with a range of problems all presenting themselves at once, and I began to feel anxious and panicked. I noticed my breathing was elevated and shallow. I drew some comparisons to the boxing ring, and recognised that I needed to regain self-control. I decided to use the method I had been taught to calm myself between rounds: breathing in for four seconds through the nose, then out for six seconds through the mouth, making sure I was filling up my stomach and using the diaphragm to exhale. I simply stopped in the midst of it all for a few minutes, concentrated on my breathing, and found my clarity of thought came rushing back. It worked, and it's something I've done in similar situations ever since.

**Pay attention to your breathing when you're in different emotional states. From anxiety to excitement, and everywhere in between, there's a different feeling to each. When you're excited, your breath will feel light and fresh. When you're anxious, it's shallow and heavy.**

My full-time gig was milking cows in the morning; I'd do that, come home and eat some toast, then head off and pick asparagus for six hours. Then I'd go and relief milk somewhere else in the afternoon. There were many days when I would be the only person to turn up to pick asparagus, so it was no surprise to later on be asked to work at night on the tractor, mulching the asparagus back into the ground. There was no point growing it if no one wanted to pick it. It was here I realised that a good work ethic was not as common as I'd thought. I'd been surrounded by hard workers all my life, so I knew no different. I understood now that I could use hard work as a way to be above average.

I began to pick up more work on the drystock farm, and began dropping milkings until I found myself there full-time.

I had been around farms and farming my whole life, but I didn't have too many farming skills. I'd milked a lot of cows, but I didn't know much about anything else on this type of farm.

On one of the first of my full-time days working there, Martyn asked me: 'Have you ever mowed hay before?'

I'd certainly been on a tractor when other people had mowed hay and I'd watched them do it, but I'd never done it myself. But I didn't want to disappoint him, so I lied and said I had. Martyn told me that the next day I had to get on the tractor and mow some paddocks, so I duly went off, and went about f**king it up for a few hours, learning the hard way how to do it.

That's been quite a theme throughout my life: being thrown in at the deep end and learning how to do it myself. One of the key elements of my success in farming has been work ethic. Right from leaving school, I had a burning desire to prove that

I could do whatever I set my mind to, and – more than that – prove my worth to anyone who doubted my intelligence. An average effort was not enough for me.

That job, with hindsight, was exactly what I needed. It was daunting at times, but Martyn was incredibly patient, shared his knowledge generously, and – most importantly – took a chance on a young fella and gave me the space to figure things out and learn some common sense. He never demanded a good job, but everything he did created the expectation of one. It's a subtle but important difference. I was incredibly thankful for the opportunity, so I worked my arse off in return.

Originally meant to stay for three months, I ended up staying for five years. Martyn approached me a couple of months in, told me I was doing a pretty good job, and asked if I wanted to stay on. I loved it, because it was new, exciting, and I was learning a load of new skills, so I said 'Yes, absolutely!'

**Give something 100 per cent effort, and you'll never know where you might end up. If I hadn't put in extra hours, showed I cared, and been prepared to do what needed to be done, it would have been a three-month gig. I was well aware of how important reputation is in farming. There was never a mention of future employment: I just gave it my all, and good sh*t happened. Don't half-arse anything in life.**

So, at 18, I moved into a house on the farm, on my own, and found myself taking over from someone who had managed that farm for over 15 years.

Martyn was great: while he expected me to take over the manager's job, he gave me plenty of free rein to learn on my own, make my mistakes, and learn from them. He was a hard boss, but he was very fair as well. As long as I was working hard, and trying, he was pretty happy.

Martyn taught me a lot of good habits, like looking after your tools, and not allowing problems to build up. As soon as something was broken, I had to go and fix it straight away.

Shortly after I started work at Cawood Farms, Martyn gave me a great piece of advice:

**'Treat everything like you own it, and you'll go a long way in farming.'**

It's a principle that's got me to where I am today, because it's an attitude that all business owners want: their staff, at any level, to show the same care and attention they do. It's stuck with me, and it's been invaluable.

## TOP PADDOCK TOOL

# Buckets of Resilience

Resilience means being able to withstand or recover quickly from difficult situations – being able to recoil or spring back into shape after bending, stretching, or being compressed.

Your level of resilience is not permanently fixed. It's forever shifting, based on the stress and challenges you're facing, and your mental capacity at the time.

Having resilience is a really important facet of a well-rounded human being. It is a word that gets said a lot these days. But what does it look like? How can we measure it? And how can we influence it?

I've found a way to be more aware of my personal resilience. I use the word 'capacity' instead.

I look at my personal resilience like a bucket. An empty bucket has the capacity to hold a lot of water, therefore it is resilient. An already full bucket no longer has any capacity, and therefore has zero resilience when more water is added. It overflows, and when that bucket overflows, your resilience is broken. Sometimes you can be an extremely resilient person one day, and then a series of events can happen, and suddenly you're no longer as resilient. It always fluctuates. I've learned that the hard way.

There are four main elements we can influence when it comes to the capacity of our buckets:

**1. OUR LIFE STRESSORS** are the water that flows into our bucket and fills it up. There's the physical stress of working long hours in a tough job, doing a big training session, or not sleeping and eating well. There might be relationship or family stress. Then a relative might die. You might come under financial stress. Suddenly you hit a point where your bucket has reached capacity and just one more thing poured into it will cause it to overflow, and everything becomes too much.

Our stressors in life are many and varied, but we don't have to take on all the stress or 'water' – some of it can be filtered.

For me, that has meant learning to let go of the little things in life that are out of my control. Don't be a people-pleaser: you can't control what other people say, or think, nor should you feel responsible for their emotions or stress.

**2. THE ENVIRONMENT IN YOUR EARLY YEARS,** and the way you were parented creates the size of your bucket. We don't get to choose the size of our bucket. But, as you go through life, you can trade up – you can grow it. You can increase your capacity through challenges and managed stress – just as I did when boxing took me well outside my comfort zone.

I feel that we are raising a generation that avoids stress and challenges. I can understand that logic, but sometimes we need those stresses, just like a muscle needs stress to grow stronger. Every so often you have to make yourself feel uncomfortable. The right type of stress – at the right time – can be a positive thing, and it is one we should seek out to help us create more capacity.

**3. DEAL WITH THE WATER IN YOUR BUCKET** whenever you can. Good habits – getting plenty of quality sleep and exercise – function like a small hole in the bucket, slowly draining away some of the excess. Talking and sharing can also help drain water away. You may have heard of filling your happiness cup – when you do that, the water for filling that cup comes from this bucket.

This is an important piece of the puzzle, and it can be as simple as you like – but with the way lifestyles are now, it is essential to fit these habits into your daily life. I've found I have to regularly make time for the good things in life. It's really helpful to understand how things like sleep, food, and exercise can either add water to our bucket or take it away. Creating a simple, quality sleep routine is incredibly helpful; not having one and getting no sleep adds a great deal of stress. Exercise is a great way to improve your sleep – it gets rid of some of your frustrations and creates feel good endorphins.

**4. OLD TRAUMAS AND PAST EXPERIENCES** are the stale old water that's always been sitting in the bottom of the bucket. That represents your traumas and past experiences you never got around to dealing with.

I've found that diving down to the bottom of my bucket and dealing with some of those early traumas has helped a lot. Some people have multiple traumas, and a lot of historic stress – I'd encourage you to try and filter through that. Often people who have been through major challenges have a really big bucket. But if there's a lot of water sitting in it from trauma and stress, then your capacity is no greater than anyone else's.

Rural men, I think, are particularly bad at allowing that water to sit in their bucket. It festers like a stagnant pond. They have a stoic mentality where everything is compartmentalised and buried.

But for the original Stoics – the Greek philosophers of the third century BC – their brand of stoicism was not just calmness under pressure, it was also an awareness of their own thoughts and feelings. They were willing to work through their problems. Yes, perhaps they did it in silence, but they still did it.

There's nothing wrong with being stoic – but not if you shove things to one side and just get on with other things. Then you're just avoiding the issue. That's not being stoic. True stoicism is awareness of your emotions. The Stoics kept journals. Show me a rural male who journals! Perhaps over time we've lost the true meaning of stoicism.

Confronting your emotions – even when it makes you feel uncomfortable – removes water from your bucket, but the challenge of dealing with it may also stretch your capacity at the same time.

As you'll read later on in this book, there have been many times when my bucket has been full. Quite recently it overflowed at a time when I was already physically and mentally stressed, and then more water came in over the top than I was able to handle. I felt an overwhelming anxiety, and I found it hard to function, let alone make important decisions. I think the bucket analogy helped me realise then that I had reached my capacity and needed some assistance to create more capacity.

I'd like you to think about your own resilience, where your capacity is at right now, and what you can do to manage it. Try to picture what stresses you are facing, and what you can do to filter them out – because you don't need to take all that water on.

Deal with the water in your bucket whenever you can, because there will always be more coming. Don't go through life with your bucket full of water because any little thing can tip you over the edge— from the kids playing up, the boss being a dick, or your car getting a bump.

What positive steps can you take today to empty your bucket? Which of the four elements can you look at now? Have you got a journal where you can write down your thoughts? This is probably one of the only times when having a hole in a bucket is a good thing. What's the state of your resilience bucket right now?

# Chapter three

# Learning to Breathe

WHEN I WAS 21, Martyn Dickie retired and decided to sell his farm. It was a sad moment for me, although I was probably ready to move on.

Most young Kiwis enjoy the 'Big OE' – a spell overseas before settling down – and my rugby had progressed so much I wanted to try playing club rugby in England.

I had just suffered my first heartbreak. I'd been with a girl for about a year, and at the time I thought I was in love, but, looking back, it was never meant to be. But she taught me a really important lesson in life and relationships – one worth mentioning.

When we got together, I didn't think I was good enough for her, and I didn't understand what she saw in me. I put her on a pedestal. Maybe it was from not loving myself or accepting myself for who I was – I was unable to see what I had to offer. Not long before we split, she said to me:

**'You can't love someone else properly until you love yourself.'**

I brushed those wise words off at the time, but they stuck with me, and a few months later it made me look deeper into myself, my past, and – more importantly – my future. I'm forever grateful she said that to me... and that I eventually listened.

An agency called Inside Running found me a contract with a rugby club in England. It was a fairly basic deal: they would reimburse my air ticket, find me a job, and pay me about fifty pounds a game.

That sounded fine to me: I didn't expect much, I just wanted to get over there and start exploring the world a little, and playing rugby in a different country really appealed to me. But about six weeks before I was due to go, they pulled out of the deal; they'd had a couple of injuries to front-rowers, so they needed a prop, not a flanker.

Instead, I went to England with an old schoolmate who had got in touch with me. She'd heard I was going over, and wanted to come. When the rugby contract fell through, she invited me to come along on a three-week Contiki tour around Europe instead. I had no idea what else to do so I went along. Afterwards, she flew home, and I had two nights' accommodation booked in London, my backpack, and no real idea what to do next.

For the first time in my life, I had no real responsibilities, no idea of where I would sleep or how I would support myself, and I was on the other side of the world. The prospect was truly exciting. There were some nerves, but my dominant emotion was a feeling of wonder at the amazing places I might end up at, and the things I could do.

Britain was deep in a recession, and I quickly found out there were absolutely no jobs going in London for a young Kiwi bloke. There was a jobs website called Gumtree, but most of the work they were advertising needed qualifications: plumbing, building, carpentry. I didn't have anything except farming, so I ended up just south of London on a Hampshire apple orchard. I figured this might be one place my farming skills could be useful.

Having picked asparagus, I thought picking apples couldn't be that hard. The guy on the phone said: 'The accommodation is a bit rough, but you're a Kiwi, so you'll be alright.'

He picked me up from the train station, and it turned out the digs were at a caravan park, and everyone else there, bar one Aussie, was either Bulgarian or Polish. They were a tough group of people, and they worked hard. I was happy to be outdoors, away from the bustle of London, and doing something different, even if it wasn't particularly glamorous.

**I didn't know much about perspective and gratitude at the time. But working alongside Eastern Europeans did give me some perspective on a different kind of tough. Comparing the life they'd come from with where I'd come from gave me a sense of**

**gratitude: they had seen war, ingrained poverty and a hard, cold, old-fashioned lifestyle without the technology I took for granted.**

I'd left my sleeping bag in storage in London thinking there would be bedding provided. I was wrong. So I ended up sleeping in a caravan with no blankets, and since it was the English autumn, it wasn't particularly warm. It was hard physical work, but the harder I worked, the better I was paid – the wage was paid per pound of apples picked.

Thankfully, the next day two young English guys, James Sadowski and James Archer, turned up to share my caravan, and we formed a friendship. There wasn't much to do in our spare time, but we made the most of it, causing plenty of havoc at the orchard and becoming regulars at the local pub. It would have been a tough gig without them.

After a couple of months, the job ended and I went back to London with James Sadowski. I stayed with him for about three months at his mum, Jane's, house in Chingford in the north-west suburbs. It gave me the real experience of England and its culture, because there were no other Kiwis in that part of town.

James was probably a little bit lost in life, just happy drinking and enjoying himself. I think his mum was glad he'd found a friend who was a little bit older. I wasn't thinking too far ahead, but I know I wasted a lot of money at the pub. I'd worked hard on the drystock farm and saved well, but I didn't come home with much. If I had my time again, I don't think I'd change a thing.

James hadn't travelled much and hadn't met many Kiwis before. He was in awe of our rugby heritage, and was really curious to learn about New Zealanders and Australians, and our way of life. Bored of our regular pub one night I offered to take him somewhere that would be a bit different to the local full of football-mad Brits. So, of course, I took him to The Outback, an Antipodean pub in south London. It was heaving with Aussies and Kiwis, blasting out tunes from back home I hadn't heard in ages. I think he enjoyed all the different people and the atmosphere as we got talking to all sorts. I was struck by the realisation that everybody had gone to England, but they were really just hanging out with the people that they hung out with at home, just in a different country. I didn't go and sleep with ten other Kiwis in a three-bedroom house or anything like that. That seemed pretty pointless to me; I know they were all having a great time, but sh*t, if you're going to go to another country, I figure it's best to immerse yourself in their people and culture, rather than just taking your own people and culture to a foreign land.

That said, I didn't actually have a job, so we went to the pub most days, but I did get to explore London with James, his dad, Chris, and his brothers, Tony and Steve, acting as tour guides.

A few weeks of that was enough for me. Motivated by the numbers clicking rapidly downwards in my bank account, and a desire for some fresh air, I fired up Gumtree once again in search of some work. It didn't disappoint.

We got jobs harvesting Christmas trees on a farm in Woodmancott, just north of the Hampshire town of Winchester. There were thousands of the things in row after row, field after field – I couldn't believe there was a place where they grew that many trees just for Christmas.

There were 18 blokes living there, and only one of them owned a car, while the farm had a van. The nearest shop was a 20-minute drive away, so we all lived in an apartment block on the estate, in a big old house with a games room and a large kitchen. A Polish couple lived there year-round looking after the trees and handling the maintenance work.

It was tough work. I remember working in the snow a couple of days. We worked 10 to 12 hours a day, six days a week. A crew came through and cut the trees down, then another crew followed, loading the trees into a machine that put them into nets and bound them up. Our job was to load the trees onto huge tractor-trailers – trees of every size from three feet (1 metre) right up to 35-feet (10-metre) monsters to be put up in town centres across England. It was like stacking hay bales – but with Christmas trees.

We worked on a revolving roster in two teams – one day out in the fields loading trees, the next in the warehouse unloading and sorting trees – then reloading trucks with orders going out across the south of England. We'd often have travellers coming in looking for a deal, so we'd sell the odd tree on the side for 20 quid. It was easy beer money.

I enjoyed the work, and one day I got talking to the boss of the contracting firm that supplied the tractors and drivers. I told him about my farming background and, once he discovered my experience with driving tractors, he asked me to return the next English summer to drive tractors during the harvest.

James and I stayed until just after Christmas, tidying up, then went back to London. I couldn't find another job – it was the middle of a British winter, and my brother's wedding was about six weeks away, so I went home with the plan of earning enough money to come back to England again.

Three weeks after I got back I played a game of touch rugby at the club and one of my best mates, Andrew Retallick, invited me to his house-warming party that weekend. The carrot was that he said I would meet his girlfriend's younger sister, Nicole. It turned out the party doubled as her 21st – which he'd conveniently failed to mention.

I fell in love at first sight, and I spent the night unsuccessfully trying to chat her up. But since I didn't have a ride home, I stayed over and got stuck into a Sunday session with Andrew and a few mates. Over the course of Sunday, Nicole began talking to me and, perhaps because I wasn't trying to chat her up this time, we hit it off. We soon began seeing each other, and it got serious fairly quickly. Looking back, I think we formed one of those connections that you can't explain. Despite having quite different personalities, we got on remarkably well and we had an immediate chemistry.

Meeting Nicole led me to stay on in New Zealand a little longer, right up until the end of June, when the harvest was due to begin in England.

**People who value themselves follow through on their commitments. If you fail to do this, you're letting yourself down much more than you are letting anyone else down. Be the person who always does what they say they will do.**

I'd made a commitment to go back, and as hard as it was to leave Nicole at the time, I knew I had to go. It turned out to be a great experience. They had all the best equipment, and the grain trailers and tractors I was driving weren't even available in New Zealand at the time. I loved it, even though I worked from 6am to midnight some days, and averaged well over 100 hours a week. The work was challenging, and I learned a lot about farm machinery and became an expert at navigating trailers down the single-lane country roads where approaching cars seemed to think it was easier to back an

18-tonne trailer up to a passing bay, rather than find their own reverse gear.

By the end of the harvest I was quite homesick for Nicole, and she seemed to feel the same way about me, so as soon as the harvest ended, I flew back to New Zealand, and found a job working on a farm at Waitotara. An old rugby mate, Sam Parsons, was converting his farm from drystock to dairying, and needed a hand.

Nicole was studying nursing in Auckland, but shifted her studies back to New Plymouth so we could be closer together.

While I worked on the farm conversion, I was offered a job managing a dairy farm, the same farm I had moved onto when I first left school where my brother Nathan had sharemilked. So the owner, Brian Williams, knew me, and knew I had a good work ethic and was relatively capable.

**There's always somebody watching. In any other situation, I would have had to start at the bottom rung of the dairy farming ladder, not at management level. But Brian had been watching me work around the district for years. He hadn't just heard about my work ethic, he'd seen it. Always behave like someone is watching: you never know what that will get you.**

While I'd milked plenty of cows, I'd never worked full time on a dairy farm, and I knew there was a lot of knowledge and skills I needed but did not yet possess.

Brian had the confidence to give me the manager's job on what was one of the highest-performing farms in the district. I had a lot of self-doubt about whether I was capable of managing a dairy farm, and I even tried to talk him out of the idea. But he saw something in me, and his confidence gave me confidence. Once again, I was going to learn on the job.

Returning to New Zealand, I realised I had visited 16 different countries on my OE, and while I had enjoyed all of them, I could not imagine living in a better place than home. I knew I wanted to settle down and think about a career. I said yes to the job. I loved drystock farming, but I could see a much clearer pathway to earning my own farm in dairy farming.

The conversion was almost finished, and I had about four months to go before the dairy farming job began, so I spent that time in a flat in New Plymouth with Nicole, which we shared with her brother and his partner. It was exciting, because I'd never really lived with anyone else up until that point.

But without a job I quickly became bored, so I returned to Steve Hartley's boxing gym and began training for another boxing match. I wasn't quite as fit as usual for the fight night in New Plymouth and, having previously fought at 69kg, I was now much bigger and went into the under-81kg light heavyweight class.

One of Steve's fellow trainers who was helping out that night came into the dressing room about 20 minutes before the fight, and casually said to Steve, 'That guy Kane is fighting is the Black Power prospect from Whanganui who's been having illegal backyard bare-knuckle fights.' Again, I was pretty shaken, but it was another reminder of just trusting what I could do, and that I could only control what I do, and not the outcome. I won the fight.

I also did a course with AGITO (the agricultural industry training organisation) to learn as much as I could about dairy cows, because I knew managing a dairy farm was a complex operation, and I needed an understanding of pasture management and herd health. To be honest, the course wasn't great, but I set about reading whatever I could to gain as much knowledge as possible.

**When it comes to learning, I consider myself an absolute sponge. Curiosity is an important attribute. It's something we naturally possess as kids, but we seem to grow out of it as we go through life. Being curious about something is the driver to become passionate about it; and then to become an expert in it.**

Nicole had decided to move down to the farm with me, so we returned to South Taranaki and, on June 1, I began work as a dairy farm manager.

The owner really believed in me, which was a huge source of confidence. Whenever I went to him with any doubts about my capabilities, he'd say: 'You'll be alright. You're smart enough, and you'll figure it out.'

The result was a lot of hard work and long hours, making all the mistakes possible and trying to learn from them. Every spare minute was devoted to cramming in as much knowledge as I could about dairy farming.

One of my big regrets in life is not asking questions at the right times. I was still a bit shy, and I didn't have the confidence to ask them. In my mind, asking simple or dumb questions would confirm to everyone – including me – my childhood fear that I was not the sharpest tool in the shed.

**The only dumb question is the one that never gets asked.**

I would consult my two older brothers a little, but given the chance again, I would ask a lot more of a lot more people – and not just about farming. But I tried to do it all myself, which is something of an ongoing theme in my life.

I certainly enjoyed the challenge. Every day presented new tests of my intellect, my physique, and my problem-solving skills. And at the end of each day, I could look at a tanker docket and see how many litres of milk had been produced, so I had instant feedback on what I'd done, and whether it was good enough.

Of course, I made a few mistakes, some of which would have cost the farmer a decent amount of money. But he was pragmatic about it; he knew he'd taken on someone very young to be managing a farm of that size, but his belief in me never wavered.

Now that I am a bit older, and I see young guys in the industry who are willing to put in the effort, I'm ready to forgive a few mistakes because they possess the attitude to learn from their mistakes, and be better as a result.

The hours were manic. June is a quiet time, because the cows are 'dry' (not being milked) so it might be a 50-hour week. Then springtime comes, and calving starts, and then it can become an 80 to 100 hour, seven-day-a-week job.

Why does it take so much time? Let me explain. During calving, my day begins with an alarm at 3.50am. Before milking, I have to go and check all the cows that are close to calving, make sure they are okay and have no issues. Because I've been asleep, it's been the longest gap since I have checked on them so it is important I get there first and deal with any problems before milking begins; for example, if a cow has encountered problems halfway through pushing out their calf, or if a cow goes down with milk fever – which is common enough either directly before or after calving. These are critical situations that I have to attend to immediately, to reduce suffering, the risk of severe complications, or death. I also walk around and note down any new calves born overnight, identify them, match them to their mother and put on a temporary elastic collar, and record it in my notebook. Then it's off to the milking shed to prepare. We have two milking herds to bring in – the main herd, and the colostrum herd. These are the cows that have calved in the last five days and are producing colostrum.

Milking them in springtime takes a little longer, partly because they are producing a higher volume of milk, so the process takes longer, but also because the freshly calved cows need extra care and attention to make sure they are healthy and their milk is of the highest quality. The heifers – the cows who have had their very first calf – are a little unsettled and nervous at the new experience of coming into the shed, so that also takes a little longer. The whole process takes about three hours, and washing up afterwards takes me up to 8am. Then I put the cows back in their paddock, and go to feed the calves, which takes about an hour; this is also an opportunity to check they are happy and healthy. Then it's back to the springer paddock to check on the cows who are about to calve, feed them out, and shift their fences so they have their new feed for the day. I take out any cows that have already calved, and take the calves to the cowshed to be checked. The cows go into the colostrum herd, and the calves go into the calfpen, where we spray their navels with iodine to prevent infection, check their identity, and give them their first feed of milk, which is very important for their immune system. Then I make sure the milking herd is set up with plenty of feed for the rest of the day. If there are no sick cows or other issues, it's home for lunch. After lunch, I check the springers again, make sure they are calving without any problems, identify any new calves – generally they are checked six to eight times in a 24-hour period – and then fit in any of the other hundred or so farm maintenance jobs and chores that need attending to. Any sick cows will get some attention – they might need medicine or different feed, or to be lifted off the ground. Then it's afternoon milking. After that, it's time to lock the herds away and feed them, and then get set for the morning. The calves get fed again, the springers get checked, and I'm home for dinner and a rest at 6.30pm. I'm back out at 9pm to check the springers again. There's every chance I'll have a cow about to calf and have to take her back to the paddock, and the calf to the shed. If something's gone wrong during the day, lunch is cancelled; there's no set knock-off time during calving, and I accept that I will finish when the work's done – not when I'm done. It's not unusual for a bad day to mean 16 hours of work – or more.

That's the routine – seven days a week for ten weeks. Every farm manages its staffing slightly differently, but on this farm, as a one-man band, I didn't get a full day off between August 1 and December 1. Anyone can manage a 12-hour working day.

But it's something different to do it every day for multiple weeks without a decent break.

The calves are in the shed for four weeks. Once they are big enough they are moved to a sheltered paddock where they are fed milk from a feeder for another six to eight weeks. They are kept separate for nearly two years on their own until they, in turn, are ready to calve. They're like toddlers; fussy with their food, needing a lot of care and attention and a very good diet.

Some of the male calves are sold to bull farmers, some are neutered to become steers and become beef cattle. Some are sent on the bobby truck to be slaughtered for veal, but that's becoming much less common. All the female calves are kept. They are usually separated from their mothers after 12 hours, which most people agree is easiest for both calf and mother.

Once calving is over, the next stage of the cycle is artificial mating, which means slightly shorter working hours, but it's a time of juggling many important aspects of dairy farming all at the same time, including animal health, mating, pasture management, silage making, and cropping. It's quite a complex time of the year, dealing with so many things right at the time when I can still experience the cold of winter, the wet of spring, and the sunshine of summer. Coming off the hard work of calving, fatigue and stress levels are high.

The tiredness post-calving is a level of deep fatigue that creeps up on me, but after so many years of it I don't know any differently. Being fit has been a huge help in managing that bone-weary fatigue, but I still feel tired. For about eight weeks at the heart of calving, my energy expenditure is about the same as someone running a marathon every day. I eat about 4000 calories a day, and towards the end of the season I start to cramp up as I move about the farm. The mental marathon is equally tough; I do the same thing, day in, day out, but it is such a crucial time of the year that can impact not only the rest of this season, but the one after, that I have to keep making good clear decisions every day. That adds to my physical fatigue and I end up feeling completely drained – mentally and physically.

I should make it clear not all farming jobs are like this. Lots of farms have rosters that allow regular days off over calving to keep people fresh, but on smaller operations that doesn't work, and being self-employed, there are no rules around time off or maximum hours to adhere to. Over the years, I've created better systems using regular relief milkers so I can finish earlier, but in that first year, if I wanted a day off, the knowledge that I would have to find someone to cover, and then pay them for it, certainly dissuaded me from taking much time away. It was hard work – but I was out to prove something. Young, fit and motivated, I was not complaining.

My only staff member was the farmer's son, who was undergoing a career change from teaching and was back on the farm to learn the job. He was even greener than me, so I was trying to teach him what I knew about farming while I learned too.

But, come the end of the season, my boss was happy. Milk production had been good, the animals were healthy, and our mating results were good. I was excited because I could look back over those 12 months and think: 'There's so much I can do differently next time to get a better result.'

I started a habit of reviewing everything I had done, and when I looked back at some of the decisions I had made, it became obvious to me that I had either made the right decision too late, or simply the wrong decision. I could see lots of areas where I could be more proactive and make better choices – in pasture management and feed management, for example – so I felt there were a lot of opportunities to do a better, more efficient job. In particular, I became aware of the chain of consequence, and how making decisions early, before problems arose, would have a real benefit to me, the cows and the farm.

When I look back over all the jobs I've done – and certainly up to this point of my career – I was significantly underpaid for the hours that I worked.

But I never moaned, because I was getting a reward that was hard to put a price on: opportunity and knowledge. That gave me so much passion and energy to keep learning and progress.

It's no wonder that people are leaving the farming industry now, or not making the progress they ought to – too much of it has become a transaction based solely around money.

There's no way I would be where I am today, or have learned as quickly as I did, if I had not done the extra work on the farm, and the extra hustle outside work hours to gain wider knowledge.

**A common complaint from farm employees is that the boss doesn't spend any time teaching them. I'd argue that many workers don't spend much time showing the initiative to start the learning process themselves. Knowledge is earned, not handed out on a plate.**

I came up with a plan to improve production and manage my time and the pastures better. Then in spring – a month into calving – it snowed, which was very, very rare in South Taranaki. The power went out, it was freezing, and there wasn't much grass.

The cows had been milking well before this, but we were quite short of feed, and I began to see cases of ketosis, a metabolic disease that occurs when cows are in a negative energy state. They lose weight quickly, and in severe cases, begin behaving strangely and aggressively.

I remember bringing the shivering cows into the shed in horrendous weather, and I had an anxiety attack.

It was a culmination of a few things: I'd had a 'downed' cow that morning, we were short of grass, I'd never encountered snow on a dairy farm before, but I knew it was going to exacerbate the feed and ketosis problems.

I distinctly remember saying to myself: 'I need to find what's real here.'

I took myself into the cowshed office and wrote down all the facts I knew about the day:

- The next two paddocks the cows would be going into.
- How much grass we had in those paddocks.
- How many bales of silage we had left.
- How much feed they got in the shed.
- What I could do to warm the cows up.
- What my options were to get more feed into them during this horrendous weather.

It was the best approach: I got everything out of my head and onto paper. I dealt with the facts, not the what ifs.

It's a tactic I've continued to use to this day. If I ever feel stressed or anxious, I take out my notebook and write down the facts of the situation. It pushes the anxiety away, because I instantly move from dealing with the uncertainties of the future to dealing with the reality of the present.

I'd had moments like these before, but this one was a real breakthrough for me in how I handled the pressure and uncertainty. I had noticed I'd begun trying to avoid stressful, high pressure situations but, after this, with the knowledge of how I could manage it, I began to find these moments brought out the best in me. High stress for long periods of time isn't good for you. But avoiding it altogether isn't either. Now I need – and look forward to – the challenge stress presents.

**My top three tips for dealing with stress and anxiety:**

1: **Breathe.**
2: **Write it down. Get it out of your head and onto paper, so you can make a clear plan. Deal with facts, not fears.**
3: **Take action. Nothing changes without actions, and if you've worked through the first two steps, you will take purposeful action. Less thinking, more doing.**

I was 22 years old, managing a farm with just one other worker, and so there was always a lot going on in my head. I was constantly thinking about work.

Over the years, Nicole often complained that when I am at home, my head is still on the farm. I think that's a common complaint in farming families. It's hard to stop thinking about it; you can wake in the night to the sound of rain, and start thinking about the cows outside, and how they are. Sh*t, most of my dreams – and nightmares – are about cows. Many a time I've woken up at night and bolted outside to check the cows aren't running up the road past my house staging a great escape.

We had powercuts over the next five days, but I kept my head, and we ended up having a great season. We set a new farm record for milk production, the herd was in good condition, and had excellent mating results, so we were set up for a good season the following year.

After that spring, I decided to enter the Dairy Manager of the Year award. With Nicole's help, I put in a lot of work and produced what I thought was a really strong presentation. I came third for the Taranaki region and won a couple of merit awards for outstanding attitude, and best human resource management.

I was, to be honest, disappointed with third place. The winner hosts a field day, where they open up their farm so people can see what they're doing and listen to the judges explain why they won. I took a couple of mates with me to the winning farm, and we all left there thinking, 'Sh*t, I should have won that.'

But the winner had delivered a better presentation than me. As part of the competition, the judges visit your farm for a couple of hours, and you have to convey a range of information to them in any way you can. He'd been more effective in getting his information across, but I didn't think he was actually doing a better job of farming. It sounds like sour grapes, I know.

**Pride gets in the way of a lot of good things in life. Life's not always fair, the fairytale doesn't often come true, and you don't always get what you think you deserve. Accept it, get over it, and move on. I held onto those sour grapes for far too long, and I never entered the awards again, despite being asked many times. If I could have my time again, I would have had another go. 'Holding onto a grudge is like drinking poison and expecting the other person to die' – it steals your energy, not theirs.**

A note here for non-farming readers: one of the key performance indicators (KPIs) on a dairy farm is the average milk solids produced per cow; the average is around 350kg. We were delivering around 460kg per cow. The previous farm record had been about 170,000kg in total, and in that second season we beat that by about 15,000kg.

Another KPI is mating performance – or how many cows get pregnant for the next season. It's called a calving spread – in the first few weeks of mating, I try to ensure that a lot of cows get impregnated, and as mating goes on the number drops. Ideally, I want them all pregnant early so we can go into production quickly; the earlier they calve, the more days we can milk them that season. So I might get 15 to 20 cows calving each day for the first fortnight.

The cows need to be well fed, so they have an energy surplus and are gaining weight at mating time, so good pasture management is imperative, and the quality of feed should be high. Cow health is also important – the chance of a cow with a lame foot or mastitis getting in-calf (pregnant) drops significantly.

I need to ensure the cows are getting the right minerals – such as selenium – in their feed, monitored by blood tests, and they are 'condition scored' which is a visual assessment of their health to see whether they are gaining weight.

The other aspect is that cows go on heat – their hormone levels rise when their egg is ready to implant – and they release a scent that leads other cows in the herd to go out and ride them.

In the first six weeks of mating, farmers employ artificial breeding – the cows on heat are selected and they are artificially inseminated using a straw. It's IVF for cows using carefully selected bull semen. After six weeks, up to 78 per cent of the herd should be pregnant, and after that, bulls are introduced to the herd for natural mating. The overall target is around 90 to 92 per cent in-calf.

It's worth explaining why having a high pregnancy rate is so important, and why that statistic causes so much stress.

In the months that follow birth, a cow's milk-production levels peak at a high point, around eight to ten weeks after calving, then naturally drop down until they stop producing.

If a cow isn't going to produce milk again, then the harsh reality is they are no longer a dairy cow, they are now a meat cow. They have to provide, otherwise we would have a country full of beef but no milk. A cow that isn't pregnant has a big financial impact on a farm business. I still have to feed them, but if I get no milk out of them the value of that cow drops in half. If that cow isn't in calf, the reality is it will probably be turned into meat. We don't want that – it's not a pleasant thing to say goodbye to them. Some people may think farmers are cold, heartless people, but it's actually really tough sending cows away to the works. However, we understand that it's something that has to be done to be sustainable. An 'empty' cow can be sold to another farmer, who may try to graze them for a year and attempt to get them back into calf; usually those are farmers who have some unproductive hilly land they can put the cow on and it doesn't cost them much. But usually, if a cow isn't in calf there is a reason why, and I don't want to breed for infertility. The day I hate the most is pregnancy testing day, when I have to make a decision on which cows to keep and which must go to the works, or to another farm. I've been fortunate to have had good results in recent years. A cow alive, and in calf, is a profit-making asset. If it's not in calf, its monetary value drops substantially. In my worst year, we lost about 15 per cent of the herd. Ideally, I want it to be less than 10 per cent.

We'd done a great job that season, with Brian's son Ross picking up a lot of the finer details of dairy farming. Everything was going well. So that's when I decided to leave.

The Manager of the Year competition made me very goal-oriented and my goal had become to own my own farm on which I could raise my kids. It was the vision sold to every young farmer, of climbing that ladder to owning your own place.

But buying a farm is really difficult without having a family farm to buy or parents to back the loan. My Uncle Ian married late in life, and had children, so any hope my brothers and I might have had of inheriting the family farm were gone.

I knew the boss' son was going to take over my job sooner rather than later. Perhaps I had become over-confident, but I decided to pursue something bigger and better paid, because that was what the pathway to farm ownership required.

I left with a great reference, and ended up moving down the coast to contract milk a bigger, 650-cow farm.

And so began one of the toughest seasons of my life.

## TOP PADDOCK TOOL

# Dealing with Anxiety and Learning to Breathe

Call me controversial, but I think anxiety is something we create: it's a state of mind, not a virus that we catch. We create it, and we allow it to consume us.

Think of it this way: when was the last time you were totally focused on doing something, but were then overcome by an anxiety attack? I've never met anyone able to answer that – yet.

In my experience, we create more problems when we're bored. Humans are problem solvers, and when we lack a focus or interest, we come up with problems to solve. For me, the best antidote to anxiety is focus. You can pull yourself out of that state by finding something else to pay attention to. Anxiety isn't present when we are doing, it arrives when we sit and think about the future and create problems out of things that haven't happened yet: anxiety is all about the future, not the past or the present.

Many times I've found myself driving down the race in my tractor and I've allowed my mind to wander on to all the bad things that might happen in the future. The fix is to push your mind back into the present – it may be as simple as looking at the next task on your to-do list to jolt your attention back to the here and now.

Another way to combat anxiety is to engage your parasympathetic nervous system through breathing exercises.

I did a lot of experimentation when I first discovered the value of breathing exercises, so it's worth finding out which works for you.

The best-known method is the Wim Hof Method.

Slow mouth-exhale for 30 repetitions, then exhale to 90 per cent and hold as long as possible before inhaling again, holding that inhale for 15 seconds.

I didn't find that it did much for me, but it may be different for you.

There are three techniques I've found that work well for me, and the one that works best for my anxiety is called the five-finger technique.

Take your left hand and hold it in front of your face, palm facing inwards and fingers spread out. Take the index finger of your right hand, and start at the base of your left pinkie, then slowly trace the outline of your fingers. As you move upwards on each finger, breathe in through your nose; as you go down a finger, breathe out slowly through your mouth.

Aim for each inhale to last at least four seconds, and always try to make your exhale a little longer. As you breathe, concentrate on feeling the sensation of your finger tracing around your hand.

I've found this exercise to be a powerful tool for bringing me right into the moment. If you can really focus on the exercise, it stops your train of thought and refocuses your mind.

The second exercise is called box-breathing. Imagine you're walking around the perimeter of a four-sided box. As you move along each side of the box, inhale for four seconds, hold for four seconds, exhale for four seconds, and hold again for four seconds. It should de-stress and calm you, and enable your pulse rate to drop.

The third exercise – four-six-eight – is similar. Inhale for a count of four, hold for six, and exhale for eight. I tend to use this one after intense exercise or stress to re-set my breathing, and calm myself down.

I began to learn about breathing when I was boxing: breathing is crucial for boxers, who exhale loudly through their nostrils as they throw a punch, holding their abdomen tight to minimise the impact of an incoming blow.

I then began to use it during a rugby game, when I was knackered and stressed, to calm myself and refocus and found it benefited my performance. Since then, I've seen both the All Blacks and the Warriors huddle together as a team after they have scored a try and use breathing exercises to re-focus themselves on the work ahead.

After successfully using it in rugby, I began using breathing techniques in real-life situations.

I now tend to use breathing techniques when stretching down after a training session. I no longer get as stressed on the farm as I once did, but I will still stop once or twice a month to do an exercise to calm myself. In the early years, I would use breathing exercises almost every day.

I made sure I practised it when I was feeling good. Because I had understood it and rehearsed it, I could reliably use it in pressure situations. Please don't try these techniques out for the first time midway through an anxiety attack.

Of course, if your anxiety can't be brought under control with simple breathing exercises, please get some professional help. There is no shame in needing to use medication when other techniques don't do the trick. You might find a combination of breathing exercises and medication helps.

Remember: most humans can only go without oxygen for a few minutes. Breathing is pretty bloody important, and most of us could take the time to understand it much better, and spend more time learning how to breathe properly.

# Chapter four

# 'Who' is More Important than 'Where'

I THOUGHT IT WAS A SURE BET. The new job ticked all the boxes for what I wanted and needed on my pathway to buying a farm. I had great expectations for what I would learn and achieve there. But looks can be deceiving.

It was another high-performing farm. It had a relatively new cowshed, and a big concrete 'feed pad' where the cows could eat supplementary feed such as straw, silage, palm kernel and maize. It was a more intense farming system, but the high levels of technology suggested it would run smoothly.

I knew the farm owner had worked his way up to owning his farm and was a hardworking perfectionist type, so I saw a real opportunity to learn from him.

It was also a career step – I went from working for wages as a farm manager to working as a contract milker. On the contract milking system, I got a slice of the milk profits. On a typical contract milking set-up in New Zealand, I'd get $1 per kilogram of milk. So if I sent 500kg of milk solids on the tanker that day, I'd get $500. The milk price can vary hugely, but back then it would have been about $5.50 per kilo, so the farmer kept $4.50 of it.

The farmer still paid most of the costs but as a contract milker, I would contribute to some of the costs, provide, maintain and fuel my own motorbikes, and pay any staff I employed. It gave me a bit of skin in the game, some business experience, and an incentive to maximise milk production – along with providing a high level of care for the cows and the farm.

But everything that could possibly go wrong did go wrong.

Two months before I began working there, I was invited along to play in a 'town versus country' trial game for the Whanganui provincial squad, in which I was up against one other contender for the back-up flanker's position.

In the second game I played, I broke my ankle, which not only ended my hopes of playing for Whanganui, but also meant I began my new job on June 1 wearing a moon boot and walking on crutches.

**The only guarantee in life is failure if you're not putting in the work required. It's important to realise and understand that you don't always get the rewards you might deserve for your hard work. Success is never guaranteed, the world doesn't revolve around you, and life can be bloody cruel. Thinking**

**that we are entitled to success – that it is somehow deserved or guaranteed – means you have a misplaced perspective on reality. Doing the hard yards gives you a chance of success. Without that, there's no chance.**

When calving began, I had just got rid of the moon boot, but I was still limping around. We immediately had a lot of animal health issues, or what we call downed cows.

When a cow calves, it suddenly begins producing a lot of milk, which requires huge amounts of calcium to produce. One of the most common cow ailments is what's called 'milk fever' when a cow becomes low in calcium, and it affects their muscle strength. I'd find them sitting down in a paddock unable to stand, or – if they could walk – they were staggering around like a drunkard. Their stomach is also a muscle, and that stops working too, and without urgent treatment they can be dead within a couple of hours.

Usually there's a fairly simple fix. But there's an industry target to keep milk fever cases below 4 per cent of calving cows. We were running closer to 15 per cent – about 100 cows. It's a lot to deal with when I only had one worker to assist me.

We also had an unusually high number of cows needing help to calve: I had to manipulate the calf into to the right position to birth, or calcium deficiency had left the cow not strong enough to push the calf out without help.

Every time I helped a cow to calf, it took at least half an hour of my time. Every time I found a downed cow, it took another half-hour to resolve. It all added up to some very long working weeks.

It felt like every day was a disaster, a constant daily line-up of problems, and every evening it felt like I had lost my way again.

**One day, an old farmer gave me a piece of advice which stuck with me and definitely helped me through the bad days: 'When you're having a bad day, it's a good idea to set the bar a little lower. It's easy to find a win for the day when your expectations are low.'**

This went against every fibre of my being, but I gave it a go and found things were not quite so bad when I compared down, rather than up.

On the previous farm, we had milked 400 cows and I had one staff member. On this farm, we had 650, but I still only had one staff member. The theory was that the technology and the set-up of the farm made it much more efficient. It was a good theory, and I could imagine if things went well, it could be done. Then halfway through calving my worker fell off his motorbike, injured a knee, and was off work for a month. I remained stoic, and tried to take it in my stride, but at the back of my mind, I wondered what the hell I'd done to deserve all this sh*t.

The problems continued into milking season. We had a lot of lame cows; I probably treated about 160 of them.

All my dreams of climbing the ladder to farm ownership were turning into a nightmare. I was stressed, feeling burned out, and I wasn't getting on well with the farm owner. We got on okay if we didn't talk farming, but we had very different ideas about how to run a farm, and he was very firm in his views.

**Being proactive is always better than being reactive. It seems to me that many people wait to react to problems after they have happened, rather than anticipating them and acting quickly to halt or minimise them. Taking early action often means a lot less work, stress and worry. Many stressful situations on a farm can usually be avoided with understanding and foresight.**

In my opinion, we needed to do something different, because what we were doing was clearly giving us problems. Doing the same thing again was going to give us the same results.

My two previous bosses had allowed me to experiment, but with this farm owner it became clear early on that his way was the only way. I was ordered to carry on doing it that way, and it was tough to take. It stripped a lot of enjoyment out of my work.

This was the first time I had experienced workplace conflict. While we talked throughout, it didn't seem to help because neither of us were communicating in a way in which we both felt understood and respected.

At the end of every season, I would review the farm, identify what had gone well, what hadn't, what issues there were (and how to fix them), what opportunities there were, and all the areas in which we could still improve.

**That year, I identified a few things about myself:**

**1: Set boundaries around how I want to be talked to.**

**2: Communicate to others where my boundaries sit, and what they look like.**

**3: Work out – or ask – how I communicate and operate, in order to better understand that, so everyone on the team can understand each other.**

This is where I first became aware of the science of personality testing, and how our communication styles and level of understanding of others can vary.

At the end of the season I did feel somewhat vindicated when the farm owner hired a nutritionist, and many of her suggestions for change matched those I had come up with during our springtime troubles.

The guy working for me had the same issues. He didn't appear to enjoy the tension of the work environment either.

We'd have 'cups on' to milk the cows at 4.30am, so I'd be outside by 4.15am, and I would get home between 5.30 and 6pm most nights. Working through the first half of the season there were many days where there would only be time for a quick coffee between jobs. I was living on one big feed at night, a quick breakfast in the morning, and up to six heavily-sugared coffees a day – hardly good fuel for the stress I was facing.

**H.A.L.T.S.**
**Use this acronym when you're reaching for a block of chocolate, or when you find yourself reacting badly in your communications with other people. Stop and ask if you're behaving like that because you are: Hungry, Angry or Anxious, Lonely, Tired, or Stressed. I find working through these words makes me stop, think, and make better decisions about what I eat, and how I speak to others. It identifies the real problem, so I can set about solving that instead of going for a quick fix.**

Once spring and mating had finished, the animal health issues began to disappear, so I thought things were starting to ease off.

Then we had to deal with a really nasty drought – certainly the worst I had seen since I'd started farming. By early January, there was no grass left on the farm, so the cows were eating a diet entirely composed of supplementary feed. That meant massive hours on the tractor getting feed to them, and the long hours continued right through summer – 4am to 6pm. It was good, at least, that the farmer placed a priority on feeding his cows, ensuring they never went hungry and buying in supplements from wherever he could. The worst thing for any farmer is seeing cows go hungry. Imagine you have no food in the cupboard to feed your kids, and how heartbreaking that would be. The cows become almost like your children, but instead of having one or two mouths to feed, you've got hundreds outside relying upon you. It's a huge responsibility caring for animals – they rely on you for nearly everything, and it's an incredibly stressful feeling when you're in a drought and you're not sure how you are going to feed the cows. For me, it's the worst pressure I can come under on a farm.

Summer is meant to be the time when I work reduced hours, do some of the more enjoyable maintenance jobs around the farm, spend some time on the beach, play a bit of sport, and have more time to relax. But that season, I – and a lot of farmers – missed most of that, and spent our time just feeding cows instead.

It was an energy-sapping year, physically and mentally. I made the decision I was not going to spend another year there. It decimated my confidence. I'd had a couple of very successful years before that, but that year was a nightmare, and it affected me for several years after.

I'd stayed in touch with my previous boss, Brian Williams, and I'd told him about the problems I was having. One day he phoned me and said: 'Look, I'm thinking about buying another farm – just a small farm. Would you be interested in going onto it?'

The deal was I would go on to this new farm as a 50-50 sharemilker. What that means is you split the milk proceeds between you equally. He'd own the land and buildings, I'd own the cows and everything to work the farm (tractors, bikes, equipment). The bills were split – he covered infrastructure repairs, I paid for the fuel and the animal health costs – and we divided the cost of the fertiliser and supplements.

It's a traditional step towards farm ownership in New Zealand; lots of people would start off 50-50 sharemilking on a small farm, then try to move up to sharemilking a larger one, and then make the leap to full farm ownership. I saw this as my ladder to ownership too, and leaped at the opportunity.

We did not have a lot of money at the time. Nicole had only recently completed her degree and started working as a nurse at the local hospital, so we were able to start saving.

The first three banks we approached for a loan turned us down. We tried to be more persuasive with the fourth, and Brian offered to talk to the bank manager himself. Brian couldn't offer us financial backing, but he said he would take his banking over to them if they supported us. The bank made it clear that we were really stretching their lending rules, but we got the loan approved.

**Attitude over intelligence, and 'I Will' over IQ. I'm fairly sure the biggest factor in getting to this stage of life was not my intelligence – it was my attitude. We can find knowledge at the touch of a button these days. Anyone can acquire skills and knowledge, but the right attitude is much harder to teach. It's increasingly rare to find people with the willingness to turn up every day and do the work necessary for success. Nearly everyone wants success in life, but not many are willing to develop the attitude to get them there.**

I was really grateful that Brian gave me the opportunity, and to this day, I still am. From his perspective, it was a huge punt to show faith in someone who only had three dairy-farming seasons behind them. He didn't have to take me on – there were plenty more established and qualified people for the job.

We wrote the budget based on my wife working full-time off the farm, and using her wage to cover our living expenses, we would plough all the farm profits back into mortgage repayments, with the aim of paying off as much as we could, as fast as we could. Our hope was that we would be there for five or six years, then move on to a bigger job.

**Every adult experiences stress. Farmers definitely do. Every day we make important decisions which have positive and negative consequences, and all of them are interconnected. It's a lot to juggle, but it is usually manageable ... until something unexpected goes wrong. In those moments, stress sets in. That's the upsetting part of stress – it's the difference between our expectations and the reality of what's actually happening. The bigger the difference, the higher the stress levels. Understanding and expecting that we create stress through this process has been the key to seeing those differences as an opportunity to show our strengths – rather than the lost opportunity for an easy life – and a lot of my stress has simply melted away.**

Two months later, Nicole fell pregnant, and we had to ring the bank and explain that we wouldn't have the income coming in that we had expected. That was the first moment that scared me – realising that we'd lost $40,000 from our first budget.

But, at the age of just 25, and with only three seasons of dairy farming behind me, we moved onto a new farm as first-time 50-50 sharemilkers on June 1, 2013.

TOP PADDOCK TOOL

## Dealing with Conflict and Different Personalities

Farmers become farmers to farm – not to lead teams of people. The classic farmer loves the work, and sees dealing with people as a necessary evil.

It was an eye-opener for me to realise that it is entirely possible to be an exceptional farmer, as one of my former bosses was – he was very successful, and very good at what he did – but, at the same time, be an awful manager of people. He had never taken the time to learn how to manage, and learn about how other people ticked. But that was not the real revelation for me: it was the realisation that I saw a little bit of myself in him. What was happening to me at the time was very similar to how I had previously treated staff working for me. I had considered myself a reasonably good communicator, but I didn't actually understand that people communicate and learn in different ways. What I considered a normal, comfortable way of communicating was perceived as too direct, brash, and even brutal by those receiving it. When my boss behaved the same way, I saw it from the other side, and that was an epiphany for me. It was apparent that I had behaved this way previously, but I had simply not been aware of it. I learned that I needed to work on understanding other people, be aware of how

I was perceived by others, and how to put myself in their shoes.

It led to a very negative environment on the farm, which taught me that culture can come from the top down.

Conflict is unavoidable. It's part of being human. I avoided it whenever I could; most people are like that. But conflict never resolves itself; it eventually emerges. So it is better to tackle it head on, and try to keep an open mind. If you understand there are many different ways of communicating, it becomes not so much about how you think you have communicated, but how the other person has understood it.

Conflict is stressful and challenging, but – managed properly – it provides an opportunity to teach and learn. I realised that successful conflict resolution requires self-awareness, empathy, selflessness, and – most importantly – understanding that doing the right thing is often not about being right. The ability to be wrong is important. I've struggled in the past with this, and argued to be right – but that achieves nothing. It's better to accept you are wrong. We humans tend to be all or nothing, and in the context of conflict, it's either all your fault, or all my fault.

It never feels right to admit to it all being our fault, so it's easier to put the blame on the other person. They do the same and it becomes a stalemate. It helped me to ask myself: which part of this am I responsible for? Then I could understand and accept some of the fault in the conflict, rather than taking a fruitless all-or-nothing approach.

I believe today's workplaces have become too transactional. You exchange x amount of work for y amount of money. Of course, that's important for both employer and employee, but it would help to reintroduce some balance where doing the right thing was once again part of the equation.

People need leadership, purpose, community and to feel good in their work environment. When that happens, there's a lot less conflict and people are enthusiastic about turning up to work.

When it was just my worker and me on the farm we enjoyed the job immensely. It was incredible to see how, as soon as our boss came onto the farm, our whole attitude and environment changed.

As a leader, it's your energy that counts. That energy flows from you, whether you intend it to or not. A positive energy drives people to buy in; a negative one cancels everything else out.

I avoided conflict with the boss. Nowadays, I would have confronted it early on and established some clear boundaries around it. By the time I built up the nerve to discuss it, I'd left it too late. By then the environment had already been established. But conflict resolution needs both parties to have a desire to fix things, and I never felt he was open-minded enough to ever consider changing. He was set in his ways, and he had a high staff turnover, year on year. I think he lacked the awareness to consider that he could be part of the problem. It's a shame, because it was a great farm.

My takeaway from this story is the understanding that leaders set the tone for any organisation, and how you speak to your team is crucial. In farming, there is a huge emphasis on the skills to be a great farmer, but sometimes we forget we also need to be a great person at the same time. You can be a great farmer but a sh*t employer.

# Chapter five

# Mental Health Needs Physical Support

THE MAJORITY OF NEW ZEALAND'S dairy farmers belong to the national co-operative, Fonterra, which sells their milk (in a solid, or powder, form) to overseas bidders.

Every month, they hold an online auction to sell that powder, giving Fonterra – and the farmers – an instant update on the worldwide trend of milk prices. Fonterra issues a series of revised forecasts through the season of what the final milk payout – or, in corporate lingo, the Farmgate Milk Price – will be. Essentially, we are at the mercy of the purchaser to set the price for our product. It's like walking into a supermarket and paying what you think the food is worth, not what the price tag says!

And in 2013, the year we bought our cows, those forecasts just kept rising and rising. I thought to myself: 'Sh*t mate, you've nailed this, you've timed it perfectly. You've set yourself up for life.'

It looked like striking out on my own was going to be an instant success.

I did love the new farm. It wasn't your typical square-and-flat operation; it had character. While the milking platform was 60 hectares of nearly flat land, it had a sharp gully running right through the middle of it, and another surrounding the boundary, some pockets of native bush and a variety of old trees for shelter. It totalled 115 hectares. It was just the kind of place I wanted to raise a family, with plenty of scope for kids to find adventure, and to exercise their imaginations. After a nightmare year, I felt like I was back on track.

Having scraped together enough to buy our herd, we had little choice but to purchase cheap cows. We ended up buying the herd that was already on the farm, paying about $1650 a head for 161 Jersey cows, then leasing another 30, with the idea that we would naturally increase our numbers by keeping the calves they produced.

From day one that herd gave us problems, which the encouraging milk forecast simply served to paper over.

We took over in the 'dry' season, the quiet time for dairy farmers. On our very first day at the farm, my first task was to move the cows from one paddock to another. Almost immediately, I noticed three or four cows with swollen udders, which was the first sign of the udder infection mastitis.

It was unusual for cows to get mastitis during the dry period, and it suggested that their healthcare regime before we arrived had been pretty slack.

The next day, I checked the entire herd and I found four more with mastitis. It was a big red flag. But I dealt with it and carried on.

Because it was my first time farming alone without staff, and Nicole was due to give birth at the end of September, I took advice to get a mate to help over calving. Taylor, an old schoolfriend, was living in Wellington and not up to much at the time, so he was happy to come and stay for a while.

Having two of us on the job made it fairly straightforward, but we encountered a lot of health issues – downed cows, cows that needed help calving, and lots of mastitis – meaning costly and time-consuming courses of antibiotics. But those frustrations were always quelled by that rising milk price.

On October 2, my first daughter, Ahli, was born. I'll never forget that moment. It's hard to describe, but any parent will recognise what I mean – it changes your life in an instant.

I felt pure happiness, but I also got that hit of responsibility that comes with being a parent. Almost immediately I began to understand my father a whole lot more.

I was lucky to have a few days off work and, when I returned, there were only a few cows left to calve and I felt comfortable enough to let Taylor go – happily – back to Wellington. I doubt he'd ever worked so hard for so long without a break.

My old bosses had always reinforced the importance of frugality. If I pulled a staple out of a fence, then I had to bang it back into shape and use it again. Want to buy a farm? Every dollar counts, so keep it lean. They also stressed that it was hard work that would get you there.

Those messages fitted with my personality, my perfectionism, and the drive I had to be the best at what I did.

But the outcome was that, over the course of that year, I became increasingly frustrated that the results I was getting did not match my high standards and the effort I was putting in. We had animal health issues. Mating did not go particularly well. Milk production was below my expectations and while, on the surface the farm was tidy, there were many underlying problems that created a large workload. The water system was struggling, I quickly found many places where the previous repair work had been sketchy, there was a massive amount of weeds (particularly ragwort, which needs a lot of work to control) and, in general, a huge amount of maintenance work for a sole operator.

The only way I knew how to deal with it was to work even harder. Looking back now, I can see that I left my wife alone in those first few months as a parent. By the end of the season, despite making good money, I was deeply frustrated.

It's a common feeling among farmers that when things are going bad on farm, they feel guilty about taking time off. I had this pull to spend more time with my young family – which I wanted to do – but simultaneously, my drive, perfectionism, and desire to succeed on the farm saw me working huge hours.

Fortunately, the payout was high – a record $8.40 per kilo of milk solid. The previous year it had been $5.84.

I distinctly remember sitting down and looking through the data on the herd. We had a really high 'empty' rate (the number of cows that had not fallen pregnant) of about 15 per cent, despite adding more supplementary feed, having extra grazing land when my boss bought another 10 hectares mid-season, and introducing more cows. A lot of the cows were poor performers, with multiple or recurring health issues.

But with the predicted high payout, I was able to approach the bank and ask for a loan extension to buy another 20 cows, and also send some of the under-performing cows to the meatworks and replace them with better cattle.

At that stage, I decided to quit rugby for the coming season so I could focus on the farm and on my now six-month-old daughter. I love Ahli, and I think she is amazing, but initially I struggled to bond with her. I wasn't sure what I was meant to feel. I definitely did fall in love as time went on, but I felt bad for not feeling that overwhelming love immediately. And most likely, it was because I was devoting myself entirely to trying to fix the problems on the farm.

Towards the end of the season, the milk price began to trend downwards, which was not unexpected. The forecast dropped down to about $7.50 per kg, which was still an excellent milk price at that time.

It was the first winter of my adult life I hadn't spent my weekends on sport. Usually I spent Saturday playing rugby, and Sundays either hungover or feeling sore. It was a refreshing change, but I spent a lot of that time going to cafés or eating Nicole's excellent baking.

In July, I went to visit my brother in Rotorua and, as I walked in, he said: 'Sh*t, you're filling out your T-shirt quite well.' I took it as a compliment, but when I went home I weighed myself. I was 90kg – the heaviest I had ever been.

I'd felt very fit at my playing weight of 81kg, but as we got into the next calving season, I realised I was struggling physically with the work. This was a new and unwelcome sensation: rugby season had usually left me in peak fitness for calving. But now I was lacking in energy and coming home after work feeling exhausted. I was slower around the farm and every task took a little bit longer. Work I had previously found physically comfortable was now a real struggle and it was really noticeable how fatigue would cloud my usually clear decision-making.

A week into the calving season, I realised I had made a mistake, and I swore to myself I would never repeat it.

That moment planted a seed in my mind. I'd extracted so much from boxing that I'd always wanted to pass on the lessons I had learned. It had been a dream of mine since my first fight to one day open a boxing gym. I now realised how important fitness was for farming, and how it could not be taken for granted. Fatigue had influenced me to make lazy, poor decisions, and had made a hard job even harder.

As the new season began, the milk price was continuing its downward trend, and soon we were heading towards the break-even point. I began working on a revised budget. Then another. And another.

In the farming community, there was a lot of fearful talk that the numbers would just keep going down.

I began to feel a lot of pressure. I was not living up to my own expectations, and without realising it at the time, my own mental fitness began to deteriorate.

I became angrier and – unfairly – I unloaded a lot of frustrations on Nicole. In essence, I turned into a dick. Stress shows itself differently in different people. For me, it was due to anger and frustration. If I had seen the chief executive of Fonterra walking down the street, I would have decked him.

**Your thoughts become your experience. Your thoughts are the filter through which you see life. The way you think about every aspect of life – the good, the bad and the ugly – directly influences and becomes your experience of those moments. It's well proven that the chemicals we produce in our body can alter our moods and mental health. They can be a cause of depression, anxiety and a variety of other mental illnesses. But the reverse is also true: how we think also causes chemicals to be released, directly affecting our mood and mental health. It's a two-way**

**street and, despite genetic variation between all individuals, we can have some influence over our attitude, mood, thoughts and mental health. Our thoughts can either be a positive cycle or a negative loop.**

I think the saving grace for Nicole was that she knew almost nothing about farming. She hadn't grown up on a farm, and her qualifications were in nursing. I hoped she didn't understand just how severe our situation was; I certainly tried not to let on just how bad it was. Her attitude was that we had a daughter we loved, our health, a roof over our heads, and we were okay – that was what mattered, not a herd of cows.

But that left me feeling like I was going through it all alone. I'd describe myself as an extroverted introvert – I like to go out for a beer and a yarn every so often, but I'm equally content not seeing anyone for a few weeks. I'd spent a lot of my life to that date alone – my brothers left home early, and then I lived on my own in my first job. I think that's typical for a rural Kiwi male.

Things just got worse. The final payout was a low of $4.40 a kilo – a huge drop from $8.40.

The worrying part was that the milk auction price was continuing its decline, creating a real fear that this was not a one-year hiccup.

I had some cash reserves from the high payout of our first season, but looking ahead to the next season, if the price stayed low then no matter how I rewrote the budget, there remained a lot of red ink.

We were also now in the trap of negative equity: cow prices often follow the milk price, and buying when prices were rising and the mood was positive in the industry meant our $1650 cows were now likely only valued at $1300. Not good when the bank already considered us a risky proposition.

When the predicted milk price fell below $4 a kilo, I gave up re-writing the budget. I could see no light at the end of the tunnel. I had bills to pay, a daughter to provide for, a long-term partner relying upon me, and I felt I had to keep everything together – but no idea of how I was going to do it. Nicole and I had put every dollar we had into the farm and I thought we had ruined both our futures. Remember, I was still only 27 years old. I was sh*t scared we were going into a financial hole we could never get out of.

I even talked to the farm owner, and tried hinting to him that he might want to buy the cows off me, and I could go back to working on a wage again.

His advice was that he'd been there before, and that it was going to be okay. We would all get through this, one way or another. It gave me a little bit of heart.

In the midst of all this, one day I asked myself: what the f**k am I doing? Why am I farming?

I'd lost all enjoyment for it. Even worse, I wasn't even getting paid. I worked out that I was paying myself minus five bucks for every hour of toil. Money isn't everything, and passion is everything in farming, but man, it's so hard to get out of bed and work all day to lose money.

What exacerbated this feeling was that, at that time, it seemed to me that dairy farming was getting very bad press. I felt that the rift between rural and urban was at its greatest. The animal rights pressure group SAFE had released a series of videos on dirty dairying, and everything I saw on the news or on Facebook was negative. The headlines about the low payout didn't help much either. I felt as if the media were adding to the pressure, and I was hated for doing my job – similar to what it must have felt to be an All Black right after they got bundled out in the quarter finals in the 2007 World Cup by the French.

That became part of my internal dialogue: why was I farming if everyone hated us?

I finally found an answer when I thought about it long enough. I was farming because, when I was a kid, I'd had the time of my life on my uncle's farm, and I'd wanted to recreate it for any kids that I'd have. I wanted them to have that sense of adventure, the fun, the ability to play in wide open spaces, and the important life lessons learned through farming. I realised that the way to get through this was to try and rediscover some enjoyment in my situation. It was time to stop and smell the roses.

With Ahli developing her own personality, I realised how rewarding it was to spend quality time with her. I made taking time off during the year a non-negotiable. $2000 was set aside for the season to pay someone to milk the cows, which covered 12–14 days' worth of work. It seemed like a lot of money when I was facing massive losses, and in tough times farmers take less time off as a way of saving money. But I wouldn't change it for the world.

**Farmers are quick to look at their finances first when making a decision, but over the years it's become clear to me that high stress levels, lack of enjoyment, and fatigue also have a massive – if less obvious – financial impact. Two grand to help alleviate some of that was money well spent, regardless of the situation.**

Most farmers would tell you they are not in the job for the money. You've got to be passionate about farming to get through tough times – because there are always some tough times around the corner. I had to rediscover that passion.

Every day, I tried to do one thing that would bring me a moment of happiness. Each morning, when I put the cows back in the paddock after milking I would go and spend some time with them and – I know this might sound daft —just appreciate them for what they were, without worrying about what grass they were eating or how much milk they were producing. I began paying more attention to some of the birdlife on the farm, and it got me thinking how bloody lucky I was to be out there working in those surroundings. Taking a few seconds to appreciate – and be grateful for – the little things I often hadn't noticed before made a difference in how I saw my day.

**Everyone needs a reason to get out of bed. I've found that taking notes, making lists and then prioritising them starts my day with purpose and focus. It's hard not to get a little enthusiastic when there are things to cross off a list, and it gives me a sense of success when I do.**

The next idea was to start taking my daughter out on the farm with me more, because that reminded me why I was doing it. It was hard to get much done with her, but geez it made me feel good. This was my real purpose and a much better motivation than the money.

Farming was in the news a lot at this time, and none of it was good. If it wasn't stories about dirty dairying, it was another forecasted drop in the payout, a mortgagee farm sale, or a reminder of the terrible suicide statistics in the rural community.

Every December, the local Rural Women's Division organised a progressive dinner. It began with a starter at one house, a drive up the road to somewhere else for the main, and then to a third house for dessert, drinks and chat for the rest of the night. A few other young couples had moved into the district around the same time as us, and we got talking to them about how good it was to get everyone together.

What was noticeable was that everyone there was facing the same struggle, but there was an upbeat community feel to the gathering.

Why didn't we do this more often? Ohangai in South Taranaki no longer had a hall or a school anymore. The school had closed a couple of years earlier, and the upkeep of the hall had become too much. Without these central meeting points, the spirit of the community shrinks, or – in some cases – dies.

Those four couples agreed to meet over a barbecue and many beers – as all good rural meetings of importance do. It was decided after drinks that if there was a Rural Women's Division, then perhaps it was time for a Rural Men's Division.

The driving idea was simply to get the community together more than just once a year.

A community Facebook page was created, and the first event planned: a doubles tennis tournament that began mid-afternoon and ran well into the night, with the final games played under a spotlight and the glare of car headlights. For a small entry fee, we got as much spit-roasted meat and food as we could eat. Despite the hard times, everyone could escape, unwind, and forget; it was only a night, but it really helped. Over the years since we've organised golf days, clay pigeon shoots, poker nights, pot luck dinners, and any other excuse we could come up with to have a feed, a beer and a yarn.

**Feel like your area has lost its community feel? If you don't have a community – make one! There's nothing stopping you from doing it.**

**Everyone needs to feel like they belong to something – a place to share, a place to feel comfortable and a place that provides perspective. You can live in the biggest city in the world and be surrounded by people, but if you don't feel part of it, it'll feel like the loneliest place on earth. A community is more than just the people in it – it's the values and spirit that they bring together that makes it special.**

Most of the events were pretty casual and organised without too much planning beyond a trophy for whoever won. Somehow I got made the president of this shambles of an organisation; but being serious, it felt to me that it had made a difference to the district, and helped everyone let off some steam during a really tough time. It was also a great way to get a few beers into a good farmer, and get them to be a bit more honest about how they were achieving success. I'm forever amazed at how much can be learned about life over a few beers.

## TOP PADDOCK TOOL

# The Four Pillars of Health

When I consider how healthy I am – physically and mentally – I always use the analogy of a table, supported by four legs, or pillars.

Those four pillars are: movement, nutrition, sleep and stress.

Nutrition is not just what I eat and drink, but also what I watch, what I listen to, who I spend time with, and what I think about. These four pillars underpin our health and wellbeing, and all facets of a healthy life can slot into one of these categories.

If all four legs are strong, everything's perfect and I feel good.

If three are strong, then my table is functional, but certainly not as robust.

Anything less than that and it's not long before I'm on the floor.

I realised that my most stressful time on the farm had coincided with my first winter without rugby training. I had failed to replace that training with any type of fitness, and, come calving time, I found that the leg that supported movement had disappeared. That put a lot of pressure on the other three pillars. The stress of a lower payout, and the farm not performing also weakened my stress pillar. There was a snowball effect – losing one leg caused me to lose the others.

At the time, I did not know about holistic wellness, and how physical and mental health are intrinsically tied together.

These days I focus intently on being aware of the state of my table legs. Life might mean that one gets a bit wobbly, but that's a cue to be even more conscious of it. And when one does falter, I focus on keeping the other three strong. When I lose the lot, I'm left with nothing to ground my health.

As parents and adults, we might always be balancing on three, but that's alright if we have self-awareness, and we know what to look for.

It only takes ten minutes a day to focus on the four pillars, an extra ten minutes to make sure you're cooking a good meal or to set yourself up for a good sleep. The simple things are best: spending ten minutes now sorting out something you are stressed about is not a big deal. It can be hard to know where to start – especially if you're presently in a position where your table is flat on the floor. I always look for the best bang for buck: what's the easiest, simplest action I can take to have the biggest positive impact? Then I do that. Go for the low-hanging fruit first – they're usually the cheapest, or even free – and spend ten minutes of time and focus on it.

A main pillar for me is nutrition (which might be more accurately called consumption) because it's not just about what we eat and drink, but what we consume through other senses.

What we listen to and watch, and the environment we surround ourselves with, plays a bigger role on our mental state than most people are aware of.

I didn't realise how the negative stories about farming I consumed on social media were affecting me. It might just be a three-minute news clip, but it could really affect my connection to my purpose. If all the stories you see about the things you love to do are negative, that feeds something negative inside you. It wasn't what I ate or drank that had the biggest impact on my health – it was what I saw on the 6pm news.

On social media, every time there was a story about the payout, there would be hundreds of comments of doom and gloom. It fed a negative feedback loop in my head. It's quite a powerful force once you unleash it, and the algorithms ensure you keep seeing more and more of it.

Allied to that were the conversations I was having with those around me. The older farmers in the district were generally quite good, because they had all lived through a similar crisis in the past, emerged out the other side, and gained enough perspective to know that this too would pass. But I think a lot of younger farmers had a similar experience to mine. And they would talk to each other. I found that I couldn't give the most negative people any of my time, because they would suck me into the quicksand of gloom with them. I could end up adding their emotions to my own burden, and I knew I already had enough to carry.

The answer was simple: turn the news off. Then the big revelation for me was when I went out and found the positive people. I learned the effect that surrounding myself with optimists could have on my mindset.

In every sh*t situation there will be someone explaining the way out and being upbeat and, just as spending time with those who were negative drew me down into depression, talking to these people would give me a little bit of hope. We are all in the same boat, but if the people around us have hope, then we're more likely to be optimistic of being rescued as well.

I didn't watch the news for some years, and I stopped looking at Facebook comments in particular. I could read a story explaining how the payout had gone down and digest that, but 300 moaning comments about what it meant – I couldn't tolerate that. I could let the facts in and filter out the opinion.

That experience has informed how I approach social media, now that I have a significant online presence. I am very aware of the vibe I produce. I want to give people a positive energy, because that's who I am. Going from just consuming social media and instead starting to create it has definitely had a major positive impact on me

I don't scroll anymore. Instead, I am selective and the people I do pay attention to are on the same wavelength as I am. They're people who see opportunities and challenges for what they are. My online environment is very different now, and more curated. There are plenty of positive, honest, informative and enlightening people on social media – you have to look hard to find them amongst the bullsh*t, but they are there. Use social media as a tool, not as a distraction.

When I began trail running, I started to look into food and drink properly. I learned quite quickly that I needed electrolytes – that was a gamechanger for me because I'd never heard of them before. Until then I'd only lived on beer, water and highly-sugared coffee.

Electrolytes are potassium, calcium, magnesium and salt. I can equate it to bovine health, because farmers understand that: for cows, magnesium and calcium are vital. If a cow is low in either of them, you'll end up with a downed cow. It works the same in cows as it does for us. The difference is that their performance is milk production – so if they're producing a lot of milk and not getting enough calcium, they'll show the same symptoms we would. They get muscle fatigue and end up not being able to get up off the ground.

When I began taking electrolytes I noticed the difference straight away, and I wished I'd known about them when I was boxing. Boxing gyms could be quite old school, so I'd have a drink before, a drink after, and in between I'd work. For some trainers, there was even the idea of deliberately dehydrating you to make training harder, so the fight would feel easier.

I also realised why I often felt exhausted – it was because I wasn't eating enough, and I was usually dehydrated.

I use electrolytes a lot now on the farm during spring and summer, when I know I will be sweating and working a lot. It's something I didn't realise I was missing out on until I stopped doing it, and started feeling a bit average – I think our bodies adjust to being dehydrated, and there's probably a big chunk of the population walking around feeling a bit below-par, and not realising that's not healthy.

So now I keep a pre-mixed bottle of electrolytes at the cowshed at all times. It might cost me $30 a month, but there's another example of the best bang for my buck. I tend to use an easy-to-drink pre-mix electrolyte.

Accompanying my drink bottle out on the farm is a snack box to keep my energy levels up. The main ingredients are nutritional (meal replacement) bars, which pitch themselves as having the right amount of protein, carbs and fat to replace a regular meal, and I'll also have some protein bars, some liquid breakfast milk cartons, and a bit of chocolate, in case I'm having a bad day.

On the farm, people often skip breakfast, because there's too much going on. They end up working through until lunch and – in the worst-case scenario – they don't have time for that either. That's not efficient in the long run. I've found a good routine works for me: I'll have breakfast at 4am, before milking, and, because I am a one-man band, I find it most efficient to work through until 11.30am or midday, and then make time for a decent lunch and to relax. I sometimes even have a power-nap before I go again. I find that I get quite hungry from about 10.30am, and I start to slow down. Lots of people try to work through to lunchtime, but they don't realise it is far more efficient to stop for five minutes, eat a muesli bar, drink some water, and then get their energy levels back to do the work more efficiently. If you're feeling buggered, and the last hour feels like a year – stop for a few minutes, refresh and replenish your energy. You'll feel better, you'll do a better job, you'll get more done – and you might even enjoy it. Too many farmers are adamant that they don't have those five minutes to spare, and that logic blows my mind. If you don't have five minutes in your day between 8am and midday, then you're probably doing something wrong. That's working dumb, not smart: it's like running a marathon but not drinking any water, or not taking an energy gel to get you through those last 10km.

In spring, I reckon the physical workload on the farm is the energy equivalent to running a marathon. I'm outdoors for 14 hours a day, and there's no sitting down. I can eat all the treats and not put on a kilo. Some farmers use springtime as a way to drop weight – some will come down 10–15 kg – and a common farming colloquialism is to say: 'That's alright, I'll lose it in the spring.' I actually want to maintain my weight, because then I know I've fuelled myself properly. Farm work requires a massive energy expenditure, and I don't think people realise that we actually need to fuel that energy properly. People tell me their biggest issue in springtime is feeling tired – but there's tired from lack of sleep, and tired from not enough energy.

Eating well, particularly in the evenings when you're extremely tired, is also an issue.

My answer to that was to get a slow cooker.

It takes a bit of pre-planning early in the day to get everything prepared. If I know what I'm going to eat, and I've got the ingredients out ready to go, I'll be alright. I can put them all together in the slow cooker when I'm having a break, so it's already slowly cooking away when I get in the door from work at the end of the day. If I see the ingredients lined up on the bench, that's the trigger for me. If they're not ready, it feels almost easier to jump in the car and drive into town to get fast food. Being planned and prepared makes the job of ignoring that urge a lot easier.

One of my sayings is 'Heat it and f**king eat it.' I'm happy with basic food. I want half a plate of vegetables, some protein and some carbohydrates. That way I'm getting all the essentials in and I make sure I hit my seven daily serves of fruit and veg. If I don't, I notice a drop off in mental clarity and performance. Good nutrition doesn't have to be fancy. Too often, it's promoted as something intricate and I can look at a recipe and think 'There's two ingredients in there that probably aren't even in my supermarket for a start.'

You don't have to spend 40 minutes and add special ingredients to get what you need.

I discovered that I didn't eat enough protein, which is surprising considering how much meat I eat. When I got into running I took a closer look at my nutrition. Now I aim for at least one and a half grams of protein per kilo of body weight. When I actually tracked the nutritional value of what I was eating, it was a real eye-opener. But when I got it right – just as with milk production – it really did make a difference to my performance.

I also supplement any meals where I may not have had enough protein with a protein shake; I think most people underestimate how much protein they should be eating if they're engaged in physical work, or taking on a big training load.

If you eat takeaway four times a week, or drink energy drinks, or a two-litre bottle of soft drink every day, you might think you feel fine, but, really, you've just adapted to feeling like sh*t. It's your normal state. It's amazing what the body can go through when it's fueled on sh*t food.

I used to fail on breakfast and lunch. Breakfast was often

two slices of toast and, for too long, lunch was six slices. I was running on fumes for a very long time.

Not until I went to the gym and bulked up for rugby did I understand how weight gain and loss actually works. The trainer at the gym told me I had to eat as much good quality food as I could handle to bulk up, to eat a lot of chicken, a lot of eggs, and drink protein shakes and I would put on weight.

Sleep is *the* most important pillar. A good sleep heals your body and refreshes your mind.

Sleep is vital to good health. If you understand how the body needs it to recover, then you'll realise its importance. I've learned I don't sleep well when I'm stressed and anxious. I never got into a good night-time routine because sleep came easy when I was exhausted – unless I was stressed. I had to deal with those worries before I went to bed, so I developed a habit of working through anything that was bothering me; asking myself what I could and could not control, what I could resolve now, and what I could defer until tomorrow.

Of course, my sleep pattern is different to a regular Joe. I'm up at 4am for milking, and I quite often go and check on the cows in the middle of the night too. I've become an expert at the power nap. Anything between 15 and 45 minutes is great. In springtime, I'm in bed by 9pm, and I aim to get six and a half hours of sleep, plus the nap – which is more difficult when the kids are around. Sleep is one of the healthiest things you can do, it costs you nothing, and yet most of us don't pay much attention to it. I do find if I sleep too much, I feel dreadful. It's all about finding that sweet spot. Create a good sleep environment – cool and dark – avoid any high GI (glycaemic index) or sugary foods an hour or two before bed, don't drink any caffeine after 3pm and abstain from screens for at least an hour before sleep. Perhaps the most important factor is to try and make your bedtime and wake-up time as consistent as possible. The moment you wake up in the morning is the moment when your sleep routine for that night actually starts.

After about 48 hours of not sleeping, people can start hallucinating. You might have heard of a lot of ultra distance runners who start seeing visions and become disorientated. All sorts of strange stuff happens. If you're only getting a few hours sleep a night, your decision-making during the day will be affected. We can go three weeks without food, about three or four days without water, a couple of nights without sleep, and only a few minutes without breathing – that's sorted your priorities into order.

Stress is one of the biggest issues we have to deal with. I believe stress is usually self-created. I've often found it comes when things to turn out differently than I have expected. Usually, it's when I've expected things to turn out easier or better for me. Imagine a day where I'm working through my list of tasks when, suddenly, the milking plant breaks down, or the power goes out. My plans have gone awry, and my stress is triggered because I know I'm no longer going to meet my own expectations. You have to accept that sh*t isn't meant to be easy. Life is challenging – life is hard – and you can't always expect it to go according to plan. Accept the imperfections of reality, and learn what you can and can't control.

As a farmer, stress is often caused by the weather. Springtime is meant to have a decent amount of rain and a decent amount of sun. It's going to be a certain temperature. There will be some wet, sh*tty days, but hopefully there will be four or five nice sunny days where the grass is going to grow. When that doesn't happen, that's when stress starts to build. In summer, you expect that it's going to be dry for four or five weeks, but you also expect that you're going to get some storms come through to bring you rain. But when that expectation doesn't become reality, that's when you get stressed. But I learned to accept that I have no control over that – but I can control how I respond to my stress levels. I believe stress is something we create for ourselves, so we can also undo it.

It takes practice – like a goalkicker kicking 50 penalties on the practice field. Practise regaining control of your stress levels, but do it when you already feel good. When Dan Carter kicks for goal at a World Cup final, he's already rehearsed it 20,000 times without the pressure, so it has become automatic. We have to do the same; the more we practise something, the more efficient we become. When we understand the intricacies, we are more capable of replicating it – regardless of the circumstances.

## Chapter six

# Home Truths

IT WAS A STROKE OF LUCK that I saw the flyer attached to our monthly milk cheque. It was an invitation to a series of weekly seminars put on by Open Country, a smaller milk processor that we supplied. The presenter, Jana Hocken, was an expert in a business technique called 'lean management'. She had worked for Toyota and as a consultant to companies worldwide, had married a Kiwi, and came here to consult to businesses and farms, including her husband's substantial Manawatu dairy farm. Her talks were all about creating efficiencies at work. She had saved some companies millions by going through their processes and cutting out all the unnecessary steps. She'd done so much for Open Country they wanted to offer the same insights to all their suppliers.

Jana asked some really tough, but deceptively simple, questions. The key question was: what do you have to do to get paid? As a farmer, I can rattle off a thousand jobs I perform over the course of a week, such as fixing fences or spraying weeds, but she said: 'No, your job is to milk the cows and get the milk into the vat.' That single task represented 95 per cent of my income. Of course, many jobs go into supporting that, but they're not the main ingredient.

She had seen a lot of farms where farmers were putting a higher priority on jobs that earned them no money. Spraying weeds doesn't earn me a cent – actually, it costs me money because I've got to buy the weedkiller, and it costs me time to go and complete the work.

She wasn't saying not to do those jobs, but to be aware of how I placed importance on my time, money and energy. I was at the stage where I would consider anything that cut my costs. A lot of general farm maintenance was deferred, which did reduce outgoings, but left me a lot of catch-up work in later years.

The other key point she made that struck a chord was to ask why farmers were trying to maximise milk production in what was a saturated market when it was essentially costing us money to produce. If there's no demand, logic suggests we should make less. All farmers had to make an early strategic decision to either reduce running costs by significantly dropping the amount of milk they delivered, or to produce the same volume of milk but reduce their costs dramatically. Both options came with pros and cons. In general, it seemed the farmers that were not in deep financial trouble took the riskier option of reducing production; those in desperate need of cashflow hoping the payout would jump back up chose to make the same – or even more milk – at reduced costs.

I'd chosen the latter option. That aligned with the traditional industry model of maximising the use of my pastures – essentially, trying to ensure every blade of grass grown on the farm was harvested by cows. Every blade wasted was money I couldn't get back. It made sense on paper, but at this stage I was under some pressure to increase my herd size. Firstly, because it would have a positive effect on my debt-to-asset ratio – diluting the debt with a larger number of cows would make things look better on the books. Secondly, I was under pressure from the owner, who wanted to see maximum utilisation and milk production.

So I increased production. We kept as much replacement stock and held on to cows to bump the milking herd up to 225. I knew, in my gut, that the farm couldn't handle that big a herd, but I didn't back myself to say no.

Looking back on these decisions certainly got me thinking about how to better manage time, money, market volatility, and even diversification. We will always be in an industry that's subject to cycles and many different influences, so finding a system that's sustainable became a key focus over the coming years.

Those seminars came at a great time for me: deep in trouble and struggling for inspiration, it was fortuitous to stumble upon this woman who was able to show me how to be more efficient and save time and money, and – as a consequence – reduce stress.

I began thinking about what I actually did all day, prioritising my list of jobs a little better. It was the challenge to my perfectionism that I really needed, a welcome distraction from the big issues, and the start of finding a solution to ease the stress.

**Jana Hocken made the point that often when we try to fix a problem, we actually fix the symptoms, or the effect the problem causes. To get to the real issue, we have to keep asking why. Why is this happening?**

**Over the next few years I kept asking 'Why?' to every problem. That not only helped me get to the real problems on farm, and in life, but I think it also helped me to develop a more open mind. It had to. When you start asking 'Why?' a lot, you have to be prepared to hear answers you won't like. I found that if I was open to hearing them, I was open to solving it.**

I realised that if I was getting paid minus $5 an hour, did I need to be outside making sure every fence post was standing straight? I was in a situation that I couldn't simply work my way out of, so maybe I could spend more time being a good husband and father.

These days I do a diagram to prioritise my working day. It's simple: there are four quadrants. Top left is urgent and important. Top right is important, but not urgent. The third is urgent but not important, and the fourth is – you guessed it – not important, and not urgent.

Everything gets slotted into one of those boxes. Middle of spring, a cow due to calve that goes down with milk fever? Urgent and important. If I don't do something, she's going to die soon.

It's important to understand that tasks can shift boxes on any given day. A water leak is important, because it means my cows probably aren't getting drinking water, but a downed cow is urgent *and* important, because I'm not going to fix a broken pipe when an animal is suffering.

Once I began to analyse it, I found a lot of things in the last two boxes that were not high priority, but I spent too much time doing. Painting a fence isn't urgent. It isn't important. An old-school farmer might make their staff go and do it, rather than let them take a break, or – heaven forbid – spend some time teaching them some new skills, because they think it is important. Because to them presentation is important and, if a job needs doing, you get on and do it. But this quadrants system makes you assess whether you are wasting time on jobs of no importance or value when there could be something more beneficial being done.

I go through this task every morning. I always carry a notebook with me. It started with making a daily note of what

I was grateful for and, after Jana Hocken's seminars, my jobs for the day prioritised.

**If you hold onto even the smallest issues, with a little time, they can feel as heavy as the weight of the world. I realised it wasn't really one big thing that was stressing me out – it was a bunch of small, insignificant issues I was holding on to, and building up. It sounds simple, but it's really important to let go of the little things. Ask yourself: does it really matter? Does it make a difference to what I want to achieve today? Is it something I even have control over?**

Over the next two years – for this was, I concede, a gradual process, as Jana had challenged my deepest beliefs – I learned to focus on the solutions, not the problems. I found that by looking at what I wanted at the end, it created solutions because I was open to different ways of getting there.

What we did to survive financially was strip away all the frills. We did the bare minimum. Maintenance was deferred for another year, abundant use of baling twine was made to hold machinery together; and if the cows or I didn't need something, we went without. We fed out the supplementary feed to the millimetre, and used the fat the cows carried to make the milk (that would have negative consequences in later years).

We use condition scores to assess the health of a cow. We would number a cow, roughly, from three to six. At six, the cow is obese. At three, the SPCA would be causing a ruckus because it was too skinny. The target for a cow that's calving is a five: a decent amount of fat on her body to ensure she has enough to start making milk once she calves. Over the season, she will slowly regain any fat she lost over calving as her milk production tails off.

Instead of calving at a score of five, my cows were calving somewhere between a four and a half and a five over the two years when the payout was low. Basically, I didn't feed them quite enough.

The long-term result was that it was harder for them to get back into calf, they generally had more health problems and their milk production was a little lower. Just like a human – if we don't feed ourselves well, we get sick more often, and don't perform quite as well. But I had no other options – there were no other levers left for me to pull. But, finally, there was some light at the end of the tunnel.

I like to consider myself as a typically stoic Kiwi male. I don't complain much, and I don't have much time for people who do.

Throughout life, I've internalised my emotions, so it was quite strange – and illustrates the level of frustration I was feeling – when I started blaming others for my situation and having a moan to Nicole about it all. I blamed Brian, the farm owner, for offering me the job. I blamed the bank for giving me the loan I had begged them for. I blamed the chief executive of Fonterra for the low payout. I even blamed Nicole for not being able to work. I look back now and think: 'What an idiot!'

I remember coming home for lunch after a particularly hard morning and having a moan about farming, and how sh*t everything was to Nicole. She simply replied 'Well, you chose it.' I was shocked at her lack of empathy. At the time, I thought: 'What a sh*t thing to say to me when I'm struggling like this!' It stuck in my mind for a few weeks, then I had to swallow my pride and accept that she was right. It wasn't what I wanted to hear, but it was the tough love I actually needed. I'd turned into a whiny, entitled dick who wasn't taking responsibility for his own actions. I'd taken the job, I'd accepted the loan, and I'd chosen to be a dairy farmer – and when you choose that, you have to take the good with the bad. I had to accept that I was exactly where I had put myself.

I had become aware that I wasn't in a good place – mentally or physically – but I felt I couldn't do anything about it.

Once I accepted my life was in my hands – and in my control – things started to change. Of course, there was plenty I couldn't control – the payout, the weather and the media –

but I was in complete control of myself. The way I dealt with 'the uncontrollables' had to change.

So I took action, and turned back to what had worked for me before: boxing.

**Whenever you get lost in life and you're not sure where to turn, then do the one thing you know will work. It's often the same thing that helped you find your way the last time you were battling. That was the case for me: boxing had saved me before, so it was the one thing I knew would help get my wheels back in alignment.**

I bought a new pair of shoes, strung up the boxing bag that had sat idle for a few years in the garage, and set about getting fit. Three or four nights a week, straight after milking, I'd go for a run or hit the bag for half an hour.

After six weeks, I began driving once a week to the nearest boxing gym in New Plymouth. I felt guilty. It was a two-hour round trip and I wouldn't get home until around 10pm, so I was missing from home for the entire evening. But I quickly discovered that while I was training I didn't think about the farm once. It was a release – a sanctuary – where I could leave the stress of the day, put on my shoes and sweat. It gave me a mental refresh and I quickly noticed that I was becoming more positive after training, I'd be a little more excited about tomorrow's work. I was letting out my anger and frustration in a positive way, doing something I loved, and I was becoming a better husband and father.

It was timely. Nicole and I had married that winter, and she was expecting our second child, my wee mate, Parker.

I was so excited to be having another child. I knew I hadn't made the best start to being a father when Ahli was born. Knowing what to expect this time, I was keen to be a more hands-on dad and help Nicole much more.

**I had got to a point where I felt that Nicole, Ahli and soon-to-be-born Parker deserved better – so I decided to be better.**

We had thrown a surprise wedding, telling everyone that they were turning up to our engagement party. With money very tight, it was the cheapest and most stress-free way we could think of, and we figured anyone who cared enough to come to an engagement party were the people we wanted at our wedding. We hired an old church, a celebrant, a jukebox, some finger food and a cake. I got a cheap suit from Hallenstein's and Nicole paid a little bit more for her dress. All up it probably cost us about $5000.

To maintain the ruse I even played rugby that day in Whanganui, so the wedding photos showed me with a few bruises on my face.

It was typical at this point that the good times in life were always tainted by extraordinary challenges on the farm. Our wedding was no different.

With all the planning done for the ceremony, and calving time fast approaching, we decided to take a winter holiday a fortnight before the wedding, because we knew we wouldn't be able to get away for a honeymoon once calving began.

All was going well until, a couple of days into the trip, a storm hit Taranaki, bringing high winds and torrential rain. Brian Williams, who had kindly agreed to shift the stock for me while I was away, phoned. It's never, ever, good news when you're on holiday and you get a call from the person looking after the farm for you.

All the water from the farm came from a dam in our main gully and was pumped from there around the entire site. We had one water source and one pump – and it was now buried under several metres of dirt. A huge slip from the hill above had obliterated everything in its path: trees, power lines, fences, and water lines.

Milk is about 90 per cent water. It takes a lot of water for cows to produce milk. They drink anywhere from 50 to 150 litres of water each day, and if they go without water for even six hours, it severely impacts their health and the quality of their output. It would be like asking an ultra-marathoner to run without water. Water is also vital as a cooling agent for the milk – the milk is at 38 degrees when it leaves the cow, and it needs to be chilled quickly to prevent bacterial growth. We literally had no water on the farm, and it was the highest priority to get something organised quickly. We tapped into a water pump on the neighbours' property and gravity-fed the water back down to our farm. Luckily, the cows were in their dry period, which reduced the water demand, but they were three weeks from calving, when we really needed a secure water supply. This meant getting a digger into that gully quickly to fix up the damage.

Murphy's law thrives on farms. Need to use something in a hurry? It'll be broken. Got a hot date after milking? You'll get sh*t on, for sure. Away on holiday? Things will be destroyed.

What I'd thought would be a stress-free and enjoyable occasion became a frantic, work-filled few weeks, trying to fix everything that was broken, and get our water supply operational again before calving began.

But everything happens for a reason, and every cloud has a silver lining.

We had a nightmare month getting the water system back up and running – all while getting married and preparing for calving. It wasn't until ten days into calving that we finally got it all done, but it gave us an opportunity.

The water system on the farm was below-standard, and had caused me all sorts of problems, struggling to get enough water to the cows and the cowshed.

I put together a proposition to Brian for a better water system, and the benefits it would provide to the farm. We priced it up and got it installed, and it was a godsend. But if that hill hadn't buried the old system, I'm pretty sure it would still be there and I'd have no hair left to pull out by now.

## TOP PADDOCK TOOL

# The Three A's: Awareness, Acceptance and Action

Good information leads to good decisions. Good decisions are usually followed by good actions. But none of that can happen without having a good awareness of yourself and your situation.

During the darkest period of life on the farm, I found myself blaming other people for my predicament. I opened up to Nicole about it, and said something about how unfair everything was, and how it was other people's fault, and how sick I was of farming. And she said to me: 'Well, you chose this.'

That really hurt at the time. It felt like a big 'f**k you'. But, as I marinated on it over the next week, I came to realise that she was right. I had chosen this. I hadn't chosen the weather, or the declining payout, but I had chosen this life, this job, this situation.

When I thought about it, I realised I was no longer enjoying the challenges farming presented to me. What had first got me so motivated about farming was that I loved challenges, and my attitude had always been to say: 'Bring it on!' I saw challenges as an opportunity to win, to learn, and to grow. But I'd reached a point where I began to see challenges as a pain in the arse; a stress that

I didn't need. That was the first step in realising that I was in a negative place, and my mental fitness was way down the scale.

Accepting the unvarnished truth from Nicole was a huge turning point. Realising that nobody had dragged me along to the bank to ask for the loan, forced me to sign the contract, or made me buy the cows made me accept that I had put myself in this situation. So what was I going to do to get myself out of it?

It gave me a sense of responsibility, and made my actions more important.

Acceptance is a huge part of moving on with life after setbacks, and it can be one of the hardest processes to go through. I see it all the time in people who are unhappy with their situation, but blame others, and are unable to accept they are – usually – exactly where they put themselves.

Yes, some of us have fewer choices because of our circumstances, but I think once you're an adult and out in the real world, you generally have a choice about what to do next. We all have different opportunities – which is a very different thing – but we do have choice.

You married that person – if you're unhappy, you've got a responsibility to do something about it. You took the job – if you don't like it, how can you fix it?

And once you accept that, you accept you have another choice: how to respond to your situation in life. In my case, it was a choice to stop moaning and blaming others, and take positive steps for myself.

Farmers are very good at working out how much feed we have, what condition our animals are in, what crops we need to plant: we can deal with and analyse all that data. But we should be able to apply the same principles to ourselves: if you are really aware of your circumstances, how you are, and how the people around you are, you can make good personal decisions.

When things begin to get too much, that's when having self-awareness can stop you before you descend down the slippery slope of negativity. It took someone else's intervention for me to become self-aware – but now it's something I do almost every day – like checking the oil, water and tyres on the tractor before I start it up for the day's work. It can be as simple as asking yourself: 'How am I?'

Often, that's the first question we ask others, but the last we ask ourselves – if we even do.

It is important to understand the things you do every day that provide you with this self-awareness and the ability to self-care. At some point we all choose – or are forced to discover – what these tools might be. I got curious about myself and I've learned a lot about understanding my own psyche: what makes me tick, which tools work for me and which don't, what I think, and why I believe what I believe. It has also given me a much better understanding of everyone around me.

The biggest lies are the lies we tell ourselves. We all have a story that we tell ourselves about our own lives. We weave in these little lies, excuses and exaggerated stories, and gradually we come to believe them. We can tell ourselves a really positive story and believe it, and that's great for our self-esteem. If we're trying to get fit, or lose weight, we can tell ourselves the little lie that we really are the type of person who goes to the gym every day, or who loses 30kg in a year and – while it's not yet a reality – if we believe that story we tell ourselves, it can be extremely powerful and become a prophecy.

But the reverse is also true and can be deeply negative: I had told myself a story it was everyone else's fault. That was a lie, but I believed it because it let me abrogate responsibility. We all do this, and now I think a lot more about the story I tell myself, because I believe these stories drive our emotions, our thoughts and our decision-making.

In that situation, I had to be brutally honest with myself. The first person in life you should be honest with is yourself. I've struggled with that in the past. It's easy to tell yourself what you want to hear. Be honest with your true thoughts and feelings. It's very hard to do, but it's worth it.

For men, pride is very often a massive obstacle in achieving honesty with yourself. Push pride aside – it gives you very little.

Instead, find a way to take yourself out of your comfort zone and really push yourself in a new way. For me, boxing and running were physical manifestations of that – they made me test my limits and strip away the bullsh*t. Another way to test yourself mentally – which I have tried successfully – is keeping a journal. Putting words to your feelings helps because it really brings clarity.

Once you've done all this, you have the third A: Action. Remember – nothing f**king changes if nothing changes. Good luck!

Don't discover awareness, take the responsibility of acceptance, but then sit there thinking the hard work is done – it all needs to be put into action.

To me, action meant simply acting on every positive thought without hesitation. When we hesitate, it gives our lazy old brains the opportunity to talk us out of it. Did you just have a positive thought? Count to four and then start an action that feeds it. It could be as simple as writing down an idea, dialling the number of someone you need to talk to, or pulling your socks on to go for a run.

## Chapter seven

# Going Back to Go Forwards

I KNOW PRETTY MUCH every one of my cows. A glimpse of a rear end in the cowshed, and I can tell you that cow's number. More than a few end up with names. My kids get the honour of naming them, so in the herd right now we have cows called Monty, Daisy, Furry and Sparkles, and in the past, we've had Snowy, Ella, Blaze and even Rainbow Unicorn.

I see my cows multiple times a day, and spend so much time with them, I do get to know them. Maybe eighty per cent are your average bovine. But there're always more than a few with their own personality and idiosyncrasies.

A herd of cows has a pecking order. They are creatures of habit, so they will walk into the cowshed in almost the same order every morning. Some refuse to go in to be milked without a bit of attention.

There are always a few who won't leave me alone when I go into the paddock, and demand to be petted. There will be a few who are shy, but curious, and will come over to investigate and have a sniff. A few will lick me. There are some in my herd that will even let my kids have a ride on their back.

Every farmer I know cares deeply about their cows: they are always the priority and we form a special bond with them. That's why, in the spring of 2017, I found myself working in the cowshed, refusing to look directly at the cows, and singing at the top of my lungs. The cows were thin, they were depressed, they had to put up with my tuneless screech, and I was filled with guilt.

I don't want you to think life on the farm has been all bad. After the record low of the $3.90 payout, the following year the payout climbed back up to $6.12 and we began to feel some hope again. There were some wins on farm too; the young animals we were raising looked very promising, and my plan for creating an efficient, resilient, and adaptable herd was coming together. I had managed to significantly decrease our somatic cell count – the white blood cell count in the milk. A low cell count indicates good herd health and high-quality milk.

I had a beautiful family, two young kids and a wife, and I felt I was becoming a much better father and husband than I'd previously been. I'd rediscovered my passion, and was enjoying living my purpose with the kids on the farm. I had hope again – and I can't explain just how much of a relief that was. We were not out of the woods, but I felt we were past the worst.

We knew it would be a long road back. We had extended our overdraft at the bank, and I took a $15,000 loan from

Brian, the farm owner. We had a couple of years of deferred maintenance to make good, but I was ready for the work.

And 2016 had turned out to be an excellent season. We had a wet summer, which is a good thing for a farmer because the grass keeps growing, so I wasn't worried about food supply, and we were able to put away a lot of silage.

As summer turned to winter, it didn't stop raining. I wasn't worried, because we had all that silage, so I fed a lot of that out to the cows, and we milked as late into the season as possible to help pay down our debts faster.

But a wet winter means the cows damage the sodden pasture by creating little footholes – in farming lingo it's called 'pugging'. If the damage is bad enough, the grass grows back only thinly, or not at all.

By the time calving began, we had a lot of damaged paddocks. That caused some stress about feed for the spring and summer and the expense of fixing up the paddocks by replanting them.

Farmers always say the weather averages out. If you have a wet winter, you generally get a drier spring. But when calving started, it kept raining, and it did not stop. A wet summer, wet autumn and wet winter had saturated the ground.

Our farm is situated on high ground which looks like a slightly sloping tabletop. A big gully runs right through the middle, with another one around the back. Usually, the water runs away easily towards the sea, and the land dries quickly.

But one day I stood in the middle of calving on a sloping paddock. It was raining very lightly, and yet water was just flowing over my gumboots. I actually had to stop and check whether it was really happening, or if I was stuck in a nightmare. Looking back, I find it hard to comprehend just how wet it got, and how many days of rain we endured without a break.

It created a huge amount of extra work in the already busy spring season – more time feeding out, and more lame cows as the water kept their hooves soft. I would pick calves up several times a day, and into the night, to stop them contracting hypothermia or drowning in the mud. Every paddock had huge puddles.

I didn't go past the farm gate for six weeks. I was just head down, arse up every day, keeping calves alive, and cows fed and healthy. I stayed positive at first because I figured the rain would stop. I had begun to see the light at the end of the tunnel, and it couldn't come quick enough after the last couple of years. I'd placed a lot of expectation on this season: in my mind, it was the year things would come right. But now it was unravelling and that light was beginning to fade.

The moment the cows walked onto the grass, they trampled it into the ground and turned it to mud. I reckon about 60 per cent of it was being lost this way. I'd try to give them 16kg of grass per cow, and – on a dry day – about 90 per cent of that would end up down their throat. That figure dropped to about 40 per cent for the two months of calving.

I had to fill that gap somehow. In normal circumstances, I would drive into the paddock and put silage and palm kernel into troughs, but the tractor made a hell of a mess in the conditions. I had no other option though, and often the troughs got stuck, creating a hell of a mess, and it was a headache getting them out again. Every day was cloud, rain and mud – the same problems on repeat.

The weight began to fall off the cows. They didn't enjoy being wet all the time either. Their ears pointed down. They were, quite simply, depressed.

I couldn't look at them any more. Practising my purpose and gratitude wasn't cutting it either, because all I could see was mud and rain.

And that's why I was in the milking shed with the radio turned up loud, singing along. And I'm not much of a singer, so that made me feel even more sorry for the cows.

It became a ritual, because I couldn't face my usual routine of checking every cow over as I put the cups on them. I couldn't bring myself to look. I'd even stopped going into the paddock to pet them. Now I just closed the gate, and went off to the next job.

That glimmer of light that came with the increased payout was beginning to flicker out. Instead, I would wake up in the night and listen to the rain hammering down, and the anxiety would flood in and stop me returning to sleep.

**Be your own best friend. I've learned a very helpful way to manage my problems and stress, and it's all around changing my perspective. There's an old saying: 'If everyone got their problems and put them in a big pile for all to see, you'd probably see everyone else's problems and take your own back.'**

**We typically see our own problems as the worst imaginable. A great idea is to write down your problems, then read them out to yourself in the mirror, pretending it's your best friend telling you their problems. Other people's issues don't seem to be such a big deal, and it's easier to offer them practical advice and solutions. Change your perspective by being your own best friend.**

It was about this time I opened up to my wife about the stress, and ended up with my head in her lap, bawling my eyes out. I think it was the first time I had cried since I was a young teenager. I remember saying that I didn't know what to do, and I didn't know if I could keep doing this anymore. I realised that I couldn't keep enduring what I'd faced over the past five years, and – for the first time – I was seriously considering getting out of farming.

I had toughed out all the previous hard times, challenges and stress. Being tough is necessary in many walks of life, but I'd been relying on it year in, year out, and eventually the well had run dry.

**Being smart can make you stronger. But you don't need to rely just on toughness to get you through when you have strategies and other skills you can call upon – that's how you leave your toughness intact for those rare times when there is no other option but to rely on. Using it to get you through all the time and in every situation comes at a cost. Toughness is a bit like a rock. You can only beat a rock with a hammer so many times before the rock cracks. I hadn't been smart. I had relied on my toughness to get me through all the hard times but it was starting to wear. Are you more than just tough?**

Six weeks into the deluge, my neighbour Phil Saxton phoned up. 'You won't believe what I am seeing,' he said.

He'd driven past another farm, which had four big palm kernel troughs out in the paddock, and he said in a 100-metre circle around the troughs, it was just black. The cows were up to their chests in mud.

I asked him how things were at his place. 'F**king horrendous,' he said, and described an identical situation to my place. Then he told me about a mate who had been trying to put fertiliser down, and his tractors had got stuck.

After he'd told me a few stories, I actually felt a whole lot better. I knew I wasn't alone. In fact, there were people out there in worse positions than me.

**Imagine how terrifying being lost at sea on your own would feel. Then imagine the same situation with mates or loved ones alongside you. What would you choose?**

**I know which I'd pick – purely for the comfort of the company. If you're in what feels like a hopeless situation, it's deeply powerful to have people around you, taking away that feeling of loneliness.**

A few days later, I finally drove into town and saw how bad it was. It takes 20 minutes to drive from my farm into town, and I pass dairy farms the whole way and they all looked in terrible condition.

That one phone call had a big impact. I began to make an effort to interact with my neighbours again after that, and the realisation that we were all in a shared predicament gave me something to cling to.

And then, sometime around the end of September, it stopped raining. The sun came out. It was the best feeling ever. I knew it was going to happen eventually, but it was such a relief when it finally did.

We had fed out all our reserves, and we had spent a lot of money buying supplementary feed. The cows were so skinny, which meant we would have poor production that year, and we would have to spend money on buying more feed to build their condition back up. I knew I wasn't getting out of the hole quickly – I had a bloody hard year ahead – but at least there was some hope.

**It's not in the middle of a challenge where you will find the lessons and growth. It's after that when it counts: reflect on what has happened, try to understand, and turn the experience into a story you'll never forget. That's where true growth and internal change is made.**

A mate down the road called one day. In the early 1980s, his parents had emigrated from Switzerland, bought a farm and done well for themselves. Every year, they had visitors arrive on the WWOOF (Willing Workers on Organic Farms) scheme: tourists who stayed briefly, and in return for a place to stay and their meals, did some work on the farm.

He had some young German men arriving, didn't have room for them all, and wanted to know if I wanted to take one in. A week or so later, they dropped off an 18-year-old German lad called Merlin. I had a bit of a giggle at his name, of course.

It turned out he had grown up on a farm, and was a really nice young bloke. I suggested to him that on the first morning, he might want to come down to the shed at 8am after I'd finished milking, and he could come and feed the calves with me and learn the ropes. 'No, no,' he said in his broken English, 'I want to come and milk in the morning.'

At 4am the next morning, there he was. Merlin stayed for three weeks, and I was astonished at his knowledge and passion for farming. At 18 years old, he could have almost managed a farm by himself. He had a great work ethic, excellent manners, and a real willingness to learn.

Each night, we'd have a beer, or a barbecue, and we'd spend a couple of hours talking about farming and life. After a tough time, he gave me some hope for the future, because sometimes on a farm, the next generation doesn't seem that interested in life, let alone hard work.

When he left, I bought him a bungee jump in Rotorua and sent him off to my brother's farm to stay, and the next morning I felt really lonely again. He'd kept me going over those few weeks with his enthusiasm and his questions about how farming worked.

**It's a lot easier to be motivated and excited about things when the people around you show you their enthusiasm and energy. Just like we absorb light from the sun, we also absorb the light of those around us.**

During Merlin's three-week stay on the farm, it had not rained. And now the ground had turned to concrete. The soil structure had been so damaged that huge cracks began to open up, and by the end of October, we were, unbelievably, heading towards drought.

The law of averages was kicking in. We'd had record rainfall for three months, so now it wasn't going to rain again. October and November are your peak grass-growing months, and by early November, we grew almost nothing. I made a grand total of 46 bales of silage that spring. The year before I had made 260 bales.

By this time I had completely lost confidence in my own ability. I'd never really known where to turn for advice, and now I had no faith in my capacity to navigate this crisis and how we would survive financially.

Over the years I had tried countless things to get the place running to its potential: different minerals and supplementary feeds, different crops including fodder beet, turnips, chicory, oats and kale, different fertiliser regimes, different grasses. On one occasion I was even talked into some snake-oil quick fix by a pesky salesman. All these experiments ended with a similar result – average production, poor mating results, and more problems and stress. I was consumed by a multitude of problems and this weather was tipping me over the edge.

It was at about this time I read a book by a South Island farmer, Doug Avery, called *The Resilient Farmer.* It was all about how he had transformed his farm to become more sustainable. The foreword to that book was written by the former All Black and mental health advocate Sir John Kirwan. I read that foreword, and a tear rolled down my cheek because he wrote it beautifully, and he summed up exactly how I was feeling. It was the first time in a long while that I had seen a non-farmer understand the pressures and the stress that farmers endured, and also saw us in a positive light. I felt we had endured a lot of negative media, and here was one of my heroes as a youngster saying that he was on our side. That was very powerful.

The book came at a good time for me. Doug talked about his depression and his battles on farming, and how disappointed he was when he could only break even. I sat there and laughed, and thought: 'I'd give my left nut to break even right now.'

It was a light-hearted moment in a serious situation. I realised if Doug thought he was in the worst spot, and I reckoned I was doing far worse than him, then there was probably someone worse yet.

**When my perspective needs a check, or I have found myself ungrateful, it has been incredibly humbling to think of those that have farmed before me— in particular Nana McCaul. I think about what the wet-weather gear was like back in her time on the farm. There was no fancy Gore-Tex for her. No motorbikes or milking machines. Sure, it was a different way of life back then, but it's always humbling to think how tough they had it. That makes me grateful for what I do have. Sometimes it's a good idea to compare yourself to someone worse off than you, or – in this case – someone who came before you.**

Towards the end of the book, Doug talked about how he got a farm consultant in to assist with his transformation. The consultant had advised the use of a software system called Farmax. I was intrigued by the idea of having a system in which I could put in different scenarios and see the financial outcomes.

His bravery in changing his systems got me excited. There probably wasn't much difference between how people farmed 60 years ago, and how they farmed 30 years ago. Most people do what their dad did on the farm. I didn't have a dad who farmed, so I figured I had always been a little bit progressive and open to new ideas.

It was time to swallow my pride, accept that I was failing – something I had never before, or since, conceded to anyone – and get some help.

Following Doug's example, I decided to get a farm consultant. It was the hardest phone call I've ever had to make.

I look back now and realise how silly that sounds, but at the time, it took me two weeks to muster the courage between making the decision and actually making the call.

We often talk about people not being able to reach out for help. I wasn't ringing a psychologist or a doctor to say I was depressed, I was just ringing a consultant to ask for guidance on how to run a farm. But let me tell you – it was hard to do.

In that 'stoic hard man' mindset, we don't ask for help and we don't admit we've lost the fight. My whole identity was based around being a successful farmer. And it felt like that reputation was shattered when I had to make that call.

**Your attachments become your suffering. We all have our own identity, and like many other men, mine was built around what I had seen growing up, and the image of what I perceived a man to be. I was suffering on the inside because of that – I had to cut ties with some of that stoic identity to be able to reach out for help. What identities do you hold on to that are causing you more harm than good?**

I ended up speaking to a bloke called Grant Lee. A farmer down the road had used him in the past and recommended him to me. Two weeks later he arrived on the farm and I gave him the tour. He looked at the cows and condition scored them at 3.8, which is really low.

When we sat down, I confessed: 'I feel lost. I've lost all my confidence in my farming ability. We haven't had a good season here yet. We've been here five years, and no matter what I change the same issues keep coming up. I know where I want to be, but I don't know what I'm doing wrong that's stopping us from getting there.'

I asked him to audit everything I was doing, and tell me whether I needed to change everything. Grant used Farmax software to audit our farm system. Luckily I've always seen the value of collecting data on animal health, supplements made and fed, pasture grown and fertiliser applications, so we were able to put in lots of accurate data and it spat out some relatively accurate numbers.

The goal was a financially sustainable business which would survive on a low payout, but also make it a job that I enjoyed. I wanted healthy, content cows and a simple system that didn't cause me so much stress, and had some resilience to mother nature.

I told him that anything was an option – I was completely open to advice. Eventually, we sat down and he said I had done exactly what I had to do to survive over the past few years; that nobody could blame me for using a bit of the condition of the cows to help survive. He said I now had to make some financial sacrifices to get to a sustainable model. It was going to hurt in the short term, but, in the longer term, it was achievable. He told me I was a good farmer, I'd been through some tough times, and I'd done the right thing getting a fresh pair of eyes to have a look. He believed that we were on the right track, but we were missing a couple of key pieces of the jigsaw.

Having Grant alongside me gave me a real feeling of relief. I no longer felt alone. I had someone there that understood the situation. He gave me a plan, which was immensely reassuring, because I really felt lost at that point.

Grant's initial advice was focused on the immediate situation, with mating about to start. It was imperative we gave the cows enough of the right feed to have a successful mating, The second objective was to make sure the cows calved next season at a condition score of five for mature cows, and 5.5 for young cows. This would require spending a good deal of our income, and then some, on restoring condition to the cows. It took some convincing to spend everything we had – and some we didn't. Over the next six months, he wanted to restore the cows' weight back to normal as the basis for a more sustainable system.

It really was all stuff I already knew and had done before – so it showed how I had become so focused on work and the problems that I couldn't step back and look objectively at the situation; it also showed how much a loss of confidence can compound and take you away from the basics you already know.

**A quote from the motivational speaker Tony Robbins is pertinent here: 'We change our behaviour when the pain of staying the same becomes greater than the pain of changing.'**

The first important element was instead of milking the cows twice a day, as was usual, we went to milking every 16 hours. It reduced my workload a little, and it also made the paddocks last a little longer. The farm is split into 48 paddocks, and usually the cows would get a paddock after morning milking, and a different one following afternoon milking. With a 16-hour pattern, they would still get a paddock after each milking, but instead of using up four paddocks every two days, they would only use three. It gave the grass longer to grow between grazings, which works well when growth is slow. In winter, rotation might go out to 110 days, but when grass grows fast, it was about 16 days; and in summer, it pushed to about 35. It also took pressure off the cows – it was one less walk to the cowshed, so it was easier to put them into an energy surplus.

It didn't reduce milk production significantly, because they get fed the same amount as before. We added in extra supplements – silage and palm kernel.

The skinniest cows in the herd went down to once a day milking, which causes them to drop production, but also reduces their energy demands. Then we dried the cows off progressively over the season based on their condition score, with the lightest dried off first in late February and the cows in better condition milking through until the start of May – a lot earlier than we would normally end the milking season.

Grant believed that if we fed the cows up, dried them off early and got them fat for the next season's calving, our projections for the following year would be very promising and we would be back to sustainability. The way I saw it, I had nothing to lose, because I was starting to crawl myself out of a financial hole, but it was either go for it or go broke, then be forced to sell.

That mating – even though the cows were skinnier than ever – was our best by some distance. Our empty rate had previously run between 11 and 16 per cent, and that year we were at just 9 per cent. That was really encouraging and gave me confidence to keep following the plan.

We spent a lot on feed, and milk production dropped, but by the end of the year I had hope, and I was excited about the job again. I had a plan to guide me, and the challenge of executing that plan. It was a turning point, and we haven't looked back since.

### TOP PADDOCK TOOL

## Problem Solving

I've often found that when I am confronted by problems, I tend to focus so hard on the issues, I cannot see the solutions. The problem consumes my thoughts, leading me to zoom in even closer on it and ignore everything else.

Think of it like standing by a brick wall. Imagine that wall as your problems, then move so close to it so all you can see are bricks and mortar. If you step back far enough, you can see over the top of the wall to the solutions on the other side. If you can see all your problems as a whole, and how they work together, you're more likely to find a solution. Take a birds-eye view and work backwards from your desired outcome, and you will find multiple ways to get there. It becomes much easier to find those pathways to success.

Where your attention goes, your energy flows. Problems are negative, and if the problem is the only thing on your mind, then it's most likely going to create a negative loop of thoughts that are really unhelpful. Instead, frame your thinking around desired outcomes. Visualising a good end result gets different chemicals going in the brain, and I've found I become much more creative because I am thinking in a positive space.

During my troubled times on the farm, I had about ten big problems I couldn't figure out. I zoomed in on each one to try and solve them individually. As soon as I thought I had fixed one, it caused negative consequences somewhere else.

There was a laundry list of issues: a herd that was performing poorly in milk output, animal health and reproduction rate; a farm system I felt was unsustainable; maintenance issues such as water leaks and weed infestations; and a high workload that wasn't allowing me work–life balance.

In trying to fix each problem in isolation, I hadn't grasped that I ought to have been thinking about the end result that I wanted – a system that produced a greater amount of milk, had above-average animal health, consistent reproductive performance and a sustainable workload. When I finally sat down and looked at the issues and where I wanted to end up, I found myself envisioning a resilient farm system that could cope with a drought, a feed shortage, or a weed problem.

I wrote down some KPIs I wanted to reach – here was my positive position, and some markers to work towards. Then I began problem-solving my way backwards from there to create a chain of events. I needed to get myself into a positive headspace where I was more creative and energetic. But it was hiring a farm consultant that really helped trigger the shift in thinking – he dragged me back from the wall and to that birds-eye view I needed. As soon as he did, it all became clear. I felt like a bit of an idiot because I realised I already knew most of what he told me, but I had been too focused to see it. Remember: being open to using other people's skills to navigate a problem is crucial. It doesn't lessen your mana to consult. In fact, having people around you that possess knowledge you don't have, or who will tell you what you need to hear – not what you want to hear – just increases your general resilience.

## Chapter eight

# Keeping Original

SO I'VE SPENT a couple of chapters going on about how tough I was having it. But it's probably fair to mention that Nicole wasn't having the best time either: we had two young kids and she was also facing some stress and pressure.

Her answer was to take up running. She suggested we both do it. I'd done a lot of training runs to get fit for boxing and rugby over the years, but even when I'd been at my fittest, I'd never been able to go further than 10km.

I came home one day, and she told me she had signed us both up to run a race. I was expecting a nice 5km fun run, but no, it was off road. I hadn't heard of that before, but when she explained it was through bush and along trails, I was interested, and I figured I'd do okay because I'd always enjoyed hill sprints and climbing hills.

It was around Lake Mangamahoe in New Plymouth, and it looked really picturesque. Then she told me it was 21km. I couldn't believe it. 'Is that far?' she asked. I told her I wasn't capable of running 21km, and if there was no way I could do it, there was no way she could either, as she'd done precisely zero running until then.

That didn't seem to deter her, so we put together a training plan and we began running. Because we had two kids, she would train first, then we would swap over. I'd finished up with boxing, so this became my replacement, and I got quite into it.

But the race itself was quite a humbling experience. We'd both picked up minor injuries in training, but kept on going regardless, and the race itself turned out to be one of the hardest things I've done. After about 10km, my knees began to hurt, and by the end, I was in agony, with searing pain through both knees and cramps in my calves and hamstrings. It was a real mental challenge, fighting those little demons in my head telling me to quit.

I've realised running is a little like farming. They both require incredible mental endurance. When I think back to the hard times I've experienced, it has often been the monotony – repeating the same old jobs every day – that really got me down and made my outlook gloomy. Running's the same – one foot in front of the other for hours on end. It's given me an opportunity to find ways to endure the suffering.

**You have to be in control of the story you tell yourself while you're going through suffering. Remember, you're telling it, so you can decide**

**whether your story is negative, or whether it is full of positive affirmations and self-belief (not hard to guess which I think you should be using).**

**Believe what you're doing right now will have a positive impact on your future. Remember other times when you've suffered, but succeeded. Replay how it felt, both during and after, and compare it to what you're going through. Think: 'If I did that then, I can do this now.'**

**Visualise the outcome, or the finish line. Imagining the detail of how it will feel to get past that milestone is key.**

It was probably the first time since boxing that I'd really been physically uncomfortable and had to push through that pain barrier. As hard as it was, I welcomed the return of that feeling. I think the race took me over three and a half hours to complete, and took Nicole about four and a half hours.

But we'd both caught the bug and set about learning how to do it properly. I realised I was running with a very poor technique, so I worked on that, and once again Nicole entered us both into a race without telling me – this time it was 36km long. Once again, I was left thinking: 'What the hell are you doing?' But once again, it was a great physical challenge. As gruelling as it was, it was a beautiful way to see new parts of the country, and the challenge of doing something repetitive like running for hours on end was just another push outside my comfort zone in which I again learned about myself and my capabilities.

At the finish line, I can remember thinking how – just a few years earlier – as part of a relay team I had run my then-longest ever run of 11km, and how hard I had found that. Back then, I couldn't have imagined ever being able to run a half-marathon – let alone 36km across hill country. It was a great reminder of how my horizons were expanding, and they were expanding not through thoughts, but through actions. It was about having a go, saying 'Yes' more readily, and thinking outside my normal boundaries about what was possible – not just on the farm – but in every aspect of life.

I found myself, then, in a really good place, having been at my absolute lowest just a year earlier. I began thinking of all the tough stuff I'd been through, and how exercise had often been the key to resolving it. And I knew I wasn't the only farmer who had found themselves in a dark place and I began to think about how I could possibly help others to find a way out.

**Being selfish is always seen as a negative, but the reality is that being a little bit selfish leads you to the life you want to live. You**

**find yourself doing the things that bring you satisfaction and happiness, and when you live that life you have so much more energy to give to others – which in turn leads you to being more selfless.**

Even though the milk payout had climbed to a level where most of the industry was back on its feet, I felt there was still a lack of confidence and positivity among farmers.

I was still uncertain about the future. Could I diversify my farm work and come up with a second income, such as an online business, or would I get out of the industry in the next five or ten years?

What triggered my decision was two young brothers who lived and worked on the farm down the road. I could see my young self in them. They both loved playing rugby, and they wanted to get better. We'd talked about it a few times. I really wanted to offer to help them to get fit, but I was too shy to ask directly.

So I had a parallel idea of offering free fitness sessions on the farm. Nicole told me to have a go, pointing out that I had nothing to lose – if nobody turned up, I could just go out for a run by myself. So I put up a post on our local community Facebook page, offering to run some boxing and bootcamp-style fitness sessions.

A few people replied, and six turned up. That was the beginning of FarmFit. Within three weeks, we had ten turning up, and I got great feedback from them.

The range of people who turned up surprised me. I had naively expected to get burly young farm blokes, but we had a real cross-section of age, gender and fitness levels. The first regulars were an older farming couple in their fifties who milked on a smaller farm. After a few months, we began to get people who were driving half an hour to join in. Our record that year was 21 people and we averaged 10 people per session.

The first season, with two sessions a week, was basic but fun. It ran from December 2018 through to June 2019, coming to a halt as calving began, when farmers are flat out and don't have the time to spare.

I spent about $1500 on some simple equipment – skipping ropes, boxing gloves, bags, mats, sandbags and slam balls – but I also innovated a little, and tried to work to a farming theme. I'd often roll out some big round hay bales, and run exercises where we had to push them around. Everyone loved that, and I soon realised that innovating with farm equipment was generally received very well and gave us something unique.

If the weather was bad, we would work out in my shed. My neighbour owned a floodlight on a five-metre pole, so he rigged that up so that on fine nights, after daylight savings ended, we could still train outside. Otherwise, we worked out in the shed with a battery-operated light. We called it 'the sauna' because it had no windows, and was dusty and bloody hot once you got going. I liked it. It reminded me of the musty smell of a boxing gym.

The concept was always about creating functional workouts that would give people all-round fitness to perform well on the farm, in a setting that wasn't your traditional gym environment.

In the second year, I began using a small horse paddock – about 100m long and 25m wide – where I built a wooden frame from some old wooden poles from a hay barn, and a piece of steel pipe to hang boxing bags. I got ten tractor tyres and a few truck tyres donated by other farmers. I also picked up 20 pairs of boxing gloves and four sledgehammers, and I mowed a 120m running track down a paddock.

In the third year, some businesses came on board with some sponsorship – my accountant Harris Taylor, and a design company, Vizlink, which was run by local farmer Gemma Adams, and specialised in on-farm communication. Vizlink also designed the FarmFit logo and custom-made a whiteboard for writing up our workouts, which now sits permanently outside in the paddock. A local contractor, Kalin Contracting, sponsored a barbell and some weight plates, and I made my own squat rack and pull-up bar. We also had some FarmFit T-shirts and hoodies designed.

I'd never trained anyone before and, at first, I wasn't particularly good at speaking in front of an audience, so I did an online personal training qualification to make sure what I was delivering to the group was the right stuff.

I got an immediate kick from seeing people enjoy themselves, and from the positive feedback I got right from the outset. I suddenly realised I had never really helped anyone else before in my life.

I'd always looked after myself and my family, and now I was experiencing this new and quite welcome feeling of doing something for someone else.

After a few weeks I began an Instagram page, and settled on the name FarmFit. I realised I was actually helping people in their daily lives, and I wondered if I could grow it beyond our local patch, so I began posting bits of our workouts. One piece of initial advice I received was to post something every day, so at first I did just that. The other reason for going on Instagram was to try and source some sponsorship, which took time because I didn't really want to charge people or, at least, not much.

We settled on a structure that was more token than anything: the first session was free; then it was five bucks a session after that, with kids and teenagers free. We also gave away free sessions as incentives during training. It's probably cost me about $8000 over the last few years, buying and building stuff, and I've probably taken in about $2000, so it's a terrible business model – but the real reward for me is in giving back to others. I get just as much out of it as they do.

**When people get something for free, they don't always appreciate it. If they pay a little, they seem more committed. 'Skin in the game' gets you past the excuses and the short-term pain to the long-term gain.**

The second piece of advice I got about being successful on social media was to make sure that I did one thing, and did it well. So I stayed focused on physical fitness, workouts and tips for exercising for the first few weeks. Then I thought that was only about half a percent of a day – there's a whole lot of other ingredients that go into physical and mental fitness, so why not put that in there too? I added stories on mental fitness, showing people a little bit of the farm and talking about the lessons I've learned in sport and exercise, and how I applied them to my business and the farm.

One of the earliest posts was about cold water. I follow an old mate of my brother's. When I knew him, he and Miah were both skinheads who went into town every Saturday night, fighting, drinking, and causing trouble and who knows what else. Now he's a vegan and has really got into photography and seems really happy – he is the complete opposite of the kid I had known. He posted about doing a new challenge every day, and one was to have a cold shower or bath every day for a week. I liked that idea. It fit with my belief in getting out of my comfort zone. I knew the benefits of doing that for my personal growth. I put up a post where I jumped into a trough full of cold water and talked about how moving outside my comfort zone had been really helpful in my life. I began getting some messages of encouragement, and I realised that it wasn't knowledge, but mindset – the barriers we create in our mind – that was the biggest obstacle for many people.

**Find your self-talk negative and demotivating?**

**A lot of our self-talk can be in negative statements: 'I'm too tired,' or 'I don't have time,' or 'I can't do that.' Try turning them into questions instead. That gives you the opportunity to offer yourself a positive answer. 'Am I too tired?', 'Do I have time?' or 'Can I actually do this?'**

**Check in with your self-talk: if you wouldn't say it to someone else, why would you say it to yourself?**

It was an awakening for me that there were mental skills and mindset tools that could be more helpful to people than just putting up workouts.

So I began delving into my past and the lessons I had learned – some of which I hadn't understood to a deep level, or how to convey them. It was quite cathartic to think back and really understand what I had been through, overcome, and learned from life. I found the easiest way to understand a lesson was to find something I already knew and draw parallels back to that. It was almost as if I could physically see and understand the lesson in something I did regularly.

A year ago, my contractor called and said he had been watching my videos, and thought about how he was applying them to his life and business, even though he's not a farmer in the same sense that I am. I think the issues I talk about can be applied to any aspect of life. We all work – it's just the environment we're applying them to is different.

**I've always been curious about people's life stories – how they end up where they are, and what they've been through to make them who they are. Perhaps it's related to my abuse as a youngster, but I've found it incredibly powerful to listen to the lessons people have learned in their lives, so I can apply that knowledge to my own.**

My mind is always chewing away over something, particularly during milking, which is a fairly mundane, monotonous task that I don't have to focus too hard on. Or I'll be out running and my thoughts drift and I'll come up with an idea. I get my phone out, and shoot a video there and then. My aim is always to get the message across in a short, sharp, easy-to-understand manner. If I don't do it within five minutes, it's gone. I'll forget what the thought or idea was. I find the way I tell myself in my head the first time is always the best version, and I find, after time, I can never quite remember it in the same way.

I think I have a straight-up way of talking that is uncommon these days. I've found that people appreciate honesty and rawness, but I also try to be positive. I feel on Facebook a lot of people complain about their lives or the government, and that was another big reason to create FarmFit: I saw a lot of moaning from people about their personal situations, with the expectation the government or someone else would come along and fix it. I bloody hate that.

I've always thought that there's nobody coming to save you – you have to do it yourself. I believe we have to take some responsibility for our own mental and physical health. You can have all the money, psychologists and government-funded services, but it's up to you to do the work.

In my own situation, I thought I could either complain and play the victim, or I could do something to help myself and others in the same boat. I was trying to act on those beliefs and motivate farmers, who'd had a tough few years, to put themselves first instead of the farm, and to get some work–life balance back. I reckon once you start taking time out for yourself – exercising, eating better and just trying to be a better person – you automatically become a better farmer.

**When you invest in yourself, you're really investing in everything and everyone around you.**

I soon ignored the other piece of advice about posting daily. Now I post when I feel like it. Putting something up every day seems like madness – I'd end up producing content with no value in a misguided attempt to stay relevant. I felt I was becoming part of the problem. I'm taking up people's time, and I am aware that people scrolling on their phones are probably missing out on the things they really ought to be doing instead. People scroll for entertainment, or they scroll for information and knowledge. I've always used social media to search out information. If there's something I want to know, I'll go find it on social media because it's cheap, easy and free. I'm not interested in the entertainment factor, but I realise it's a part of engaging people.

Before I post, I ask myself: 'Am I helping people, or am I just sucking up their time and energy?' I don't want to put up posts that aren't high value, or aren't going to be of benefit to anyone. I could maximise my audience by producing more content, but that's not my main motivation and it doesn't align with my values.

My online following has grown to about 15,000 people. When I first began posting on social media I imagined that 500 followers would be an amazing result. 15,000 is mindblowing –

and it just keeps growing. While the majority are rural New Zealanders, we've really expanded beyond our target market and got a sizable amount of city dwellers and followers from the US, the UK and Australia. A lot of my posts have had over 100,000 views, and many have had around 50,000 views.

I'm often told I am a natural at speaking on camera, or in person, as if it's a gift I was born with. It's not. If people could see my first few videos, or more pertinently, some of my early videos – which never got posted because they were awful – they would realise I am far from a natural talent. I still feel quite uncomfortable – and it took me ages to get up the courage to start making videos where I spoke directly to the camera. But I did it often, and now I am better at it.

**Do the Reps: practise, experiment, and understand what you're doing. Sport and training are an excellent practice environment for many of the tips and tools in this book.**

**Whether it's a physical or a mental skill, you've got to keep practising it before you need it. Don't read how to do breathing exercises, and then expect to nail them while in the middle of an anxiety attack.**

The result of that growth has been a steady and increasing flow of people responding directly to me, wanting help or advice. I get messages from people who aren't in a good place in their life, and are struggling with their mental health or their work.

My response is to get curious about their lives. I start a conversation to try and understand where they are at, and what's got them there. I talk to some on the phone rather than messaging. I try to understand and empathise, and hopefully lift some weight from their shoulders – I know that it would help for me. I'm not there to fix their problems, but I am there to listen and, if they want me to, I will give them my two cents on what they might do to move forward, or suggest someone to go to who might be able to help.

I might speak to a couple of people a week, then hear nothing for three weeks. I think it depends on whether I've posted something that has really resonated with people. I've got enough of an audience now that I think every post finds someone for whom it really hits home.

I understand, particularly for the men, how hard it has been for them to contact me, so I appreciate their bravery in reaching out, and I hope I've been some small help.

It also helps me, and I can't thank them enough. There have been times when I've been close to throwing it all away, then I get a message and I think I have to keep going; that I am on the right track. Every time I've been close to quitting because I feel like I've given out a lot and not got a lot back, a message out of the blue will make it all feel worthwhile again.

It could simply say: 'Hey, mate, been listening to your videos and watching your stuff for quite a long time. I really enjoy them' and it really makes me smile. It puts a piece of wood on my fire and keeps it burning, because it speaks to a newly discovered purpose: to help people.

## TOP PADDOCK TOOL

# Physical and Mental Fitness

If I approached the group that turn up regularly to my place for FarmFit sessions and asked them: 'Are you fit?' the majority of them would say no. They'd be wrong, of course. Most Kiwis would say that, because nobody wants to be the big-noter in the group.

There's the odd person who backs themselves and says yes, and there'll be a few in the middle ground who aren't really sure what to say.

I think the same applies with mental health. It feels as if the only answers you're permitted to give are that you're either mentally unwell, or you're 'normal'.

But there is not a 'yes' or 'no' answer to either question. Everyone is somewhere on the scale from 1 to 100. If you're Usain Bolt or Richie McCaw, then maybe you're at 100, or somewhere close to it. Someone who is bedridden with a multitude of health conditions might be a 1, or they could feel like they're at 50, all things considered.

Everyone else is somewhere in between, and their number is always fluctuating. If I look back over my own mental and physical health at different times of my life, it's been a constant ebb and flow.

Even world-class athletes aren't at 100 all the time. They might aim to peak at 100 for a major event, then bring it back down, because it's not sustainable to stay at that level all the time. It's important for people to grasp the idea that there are going to be times in your life when your mental health might dip down to 40, 30, or even 20.

If you become accustomed to seeing it as a scale – rather than a yes/no answer – then you can gain an understanding that it's actually okay to be a little off-kilter, and work out what's needed to lift that number back up. I'd consider that as a more effective and positive way to consider things than labelling yourself physically or mentally healthy or unhealthy.

I like the terms 'mental fitness' and 'physical fitness' because there are so many parallels between the two, and I believe the same skillset is required to improve both.

If you consider your health as a number that can change, then it's easier to accept you will have bad days and good days.

You can be at your peak fitness – just like I was when I was boxing – but it's very easy to get stale, over-train, and begin to dip. You want to get to a high level, and once you've performed for your peak event, bring it gently down again to recover.

It would be good for people to realise it's okay to not be a 'yes', but it doesn't mean you're a 'no' either, and it's okay to be on that scale between 20 and 80, live there comfortably, and move up and down as you need to. Everyone will have a bottom and top number that they normally float between that's unique to them. We just need to recognise what they are and – more importantly – recognise when we go outside those normal parameters.

If you're in a place where you're struggling and your number is low, then you need to understand it takes time to get fit. Writing this chapter, I was in training for an ultra-marathon. The first month of training was awful. It wasn't until I'd got some base fitness going that the runs began to feel better, and I felt a noticeable improvement in performance. The work you do today isn't for today, it's for next week or next month.

The same with mental fitness. That journal entry you write today may not deliver a noticeable improvement right now, but if you write consistently every day, in three weeks' time you'll find yourself in a very different place.

One run doesn't get you fit, but ten runs gets you on the pathway there. Consistently doing little things for your mental fitness will slowly deliver you to a better place.

Then you have to do some work to maintain it. To maintain my present level of physical fitness would probably require one run a week and one strength session. I won't gain anything, but I probably won't lose anything.

So when you're feeling good, doing some work helps to maintain that feeling a little longer. Try to find a plateau up there, rather than dipping straight back down again. You have to be proactive to achieve this.

Consider your mood like the swell of the ocean – rolling up and down.

Some days, we just wake up and we're not so good. We feel low on energy, low on mood, and we think negative thoughts. We all have those days. We also have those days where everything makes us smile and the world is a great place to be. Some people's waves are very deep like the Southern Ocean in a gale-force wind; some people's are a gentle day where the sea is like a sheet of glass.

I've always believed when you're riding the crest of a big wave, you can do something to make sure you don't dip deep into the swell next time. Make those waves a bit smoother and you're less likely to get consumed by rough times.

FarmFit helped smooth those waves for me. It put me under a bit of stress and pressure at a time when I was in a good place, and I knew that would give me useful practice for when I am not in a good place.

Every spring and summer when I worked on the drystock farm, I had to spray weedkiller on the ragwort growing on the hills. It's a bloody hard job: a fortnight of tramping around 60 hectares of hill country with a 15kg backpack. It got me fit and strong, but it was tough work in the heat. My boss told me the story of when he first took over the farm. The ragwort was thick and widespread. He'd managed, over three decades, to reduce it to a manageable level. But every year, I had to cover that ground to spray the remaining baby ragwort before it flowered and blew its seed everywhere. 'Over 30 years, I've managed to get it from a really bad problem to a problem that's heaps easier to manage,' he said. 'But whoever is here for the next 30 years will still have to spray it, because the seeds stay in the soil for so long.'

But he was stoic about it. 'This is the rent I pay,' he said. 'I've got a beautiful farm here, it grows heaps of grass. But this is the rent I've got to pay every year – to go out and spray that ragwort.' Then he paused for a second, and thought about it, and added: 'Well, you do, because you're young.'

If you don't pay the rent, then the debt collector will turn up eventually. You might end up with a health problem. The pandemic has shown that people with pre-existing medical conditions are more at risk of COVID-19. But I haven't seen a government anywhere talking about – let alone implementing – a programme to lift people's basic immunity. I thought it was absolute madness to see people being enticed to get a COVID-19 vaccination by offering them a free pack of fast food. In my opinion they don't need fast food – they need fruit and vegetables, good nutrition, and the knowledge to go with it.

I view our bodies as this amazing vessel that can do amazing things, but it takes a little bit of maintenance. Even if you don't like your particular vessel, you have to pay that rent. But there are a lot of people in society who, I believe, are not paying their rent.

Our mental and physical health are intrinsically linked. Good mental health needs great physical support: you can't be in a good space mentally without doing physical activities to create that space.

Recently I've found it a lot easier to replace the phrase 'mental health' with 'mental fitness'. It changed my perspective to something that's easier to be aware of, to understand, and to work on improving.

## Chapter nine

# FarmFit at Home

I SEE A PARALLEL between a training programme – regardless of whether your target is weight loss, an athletic discipline, body composition change, or just getting fitter for farming or life – and building a house.

Houses, no matter what they finally end up looking like, usually have very similar foundations.

You can't build a solid house on weak foundations; the same goes for your body.

Start your training with a solid foundation. That foundation should be the same for everyone – whether you're a body builder, a rugby player, or an absolute novice.

The Russians came up with the term 'general physical preparedness' to describe the way they train their kids to be able to turn their hand to anything. Kids don't know what they are going to be good at – so it's good practice to get them to try out a wide range of sporting activities.

Some people look at swimmers, see their broad, powerful shoulders and long lean bodies, and presume that's a physique forged by swimming. I think the opposite is true – we are looking at someone who has discovered the sporting discipline that best suits their body type.

General physical preparedness teaches good all-rounders. The foundation comes from big movements – think of the things kids would do – lots of pushing and pulling things, jumping over things, and movements that allow kids to transition into specific activities with ease.

Building a good training foundation involves movements like squats, deadlifts, push-ups and pull-ups, and carrying things are great for strength. For a good aerobic base, your steady state (aerobic) energy system needs to be built first, so reps at that stage are high, and your load is low. There should be a component that challenges your stability and how you move your body through space. A strong focus on technique with all movements, along with something like a one-legged deadlift or a lunge that transitions into a high-knee lift, can build awareness of how your body moves and functions, and ensures it is moving properly, not just taking the easiest route.

FarmFit is principally based on that initial phase of training – getting people to a state of general physical preparedness. We do a lot of big movements, and a lot of carrying awkward and unevenly weighted things, because out on the farm, you don't sit at a weights bench, you move through time and space, and often eccentrically: when you're carrying an animal, for example, you know that it will shift and fidget in your arms.

Some basic exercises we love at this stage are flipping truck and tractor tyres – a good general movement that carries over into real life and sport – and the farmer's carry, where you carry a bucket or container filled with water or sand in each hand and walk with them. That's a great functional movement good for posture, core strength and leg strength. Because we are on a farm, we use drench containers filled with water, sand or cement.

You typically spend between four and eight weeks in that foundational stage. As you progress, you can increase the load or repetitions you use for your strength work, and for your running.

Aerobic exercise is often called 'cardio' – it's when your heart pumps oxegenated blood to your muscles so they can burn fuel and move. Anaerobic exercise is short, intense physical activity that is fuelled by energy sources in the muscles being used so you can only do anaerobic exercise for a short amount of time.

Running aerobically, without getting into smartwatches and heart-rate sensors, is whether you can still string a sentence together without gasping for breath. Anaerobic is the feeling when you're running so hard that you can't breathe, your lungs start to burn and your muscles become heavy with lactic acid. Our aim is to stay in that aerobic zone and run further.

Everyone, from the complete novice to the elite athlete, should also spend time in the aerobic phase. Starting with light loads and high reps is important for building strength in your tendons and ligaments. If you've ever cut up an animal, you can see that these body parts are not like our other muscles – hard and stringy, with less blood flow – they take longer to get stronger. These lighter loads allow time for them to adapt.

In this phase of training, a circuit – or to use a Crossfit term, an AMRAP (As Many Rounds As Possible) – works well.

**Here's an example based on a five-workout week:**

**Monday:** Run/walk at a steady state – aim to be able to string sentences together for the whole run. If you get out of breath, don't worry, drop down to a walk until you can run again. Your starting point for distance will be very individual – but a good target at this pace should be 30 minutes, working your way up to an hour.

**Tuesday:** Circuit. We're aiming to keep the heart rate and breathing consistent, so rest as needed in between exercises and rounds. Pick a regression or progression (a simplified version, or a harder version) that allows you to complete 12 to 16 reps, and progress over the weeks, up to 28 reps before increasing the load/weight.

Here's a typical circuit:

- Pushups
- Squats
- Plank hold

- Lunge to high knee
- One of the following: a bent-over row; pull-up or inverted row; prone cobra
- Deadlift
- Farmers carry – aim for 50 metres plus
- Ground to overhead – pick something up, lift it to your chest, then shoulder-press it over your head

Repeat for two to four rounds, with rests as required

**Wednesday:** Rest

**Thursday:** Two separate AMRAP to be completed for 12 minutes each:

A) 16 Squats

B) 60m farmers carry

C) 16 pushups

A) 30m walking lunge

B) 8-per-leg plank leg raise

C) 8 chest-to-ground burpees

**Friday:** Repeat Tuesday's circuit

**Saturday:** Repeat Monday's steady-state activity

**Sunday:** Rest

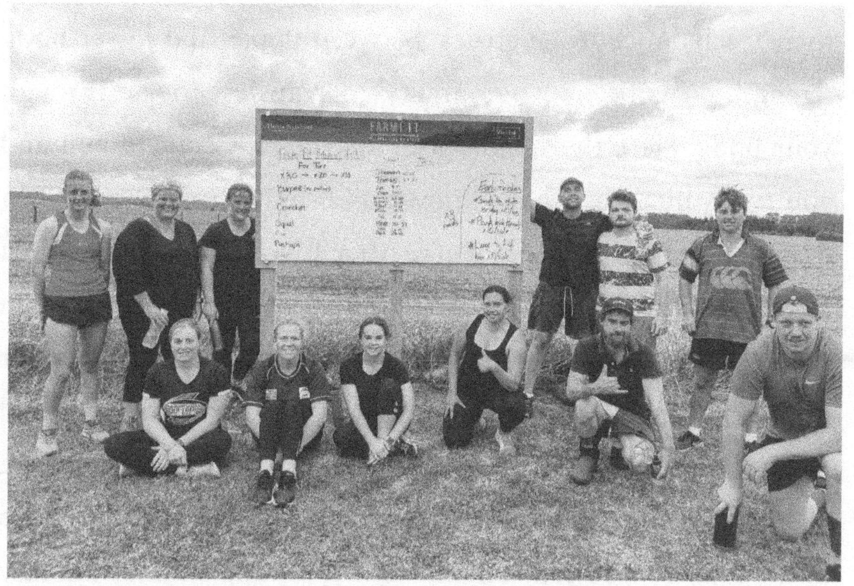

*Farm Fit crew with our new outdoor whiteboard, after a workout.*

The next phase of training is where you become more specific. In the house analogy, it's when you put up the framing and decide how many bedrooms and bathrooms it will have. Start building muscle mass, and change or add movements to suit your end goal. For farmers seeking on-farm fitness, I would not get too specific here – staying general is fine, but perhaps consider a focus on core rotational movements, back strength, shoulders and legs.

Identify the areas of your body that will come under the most load. For runners, a lot of load goes through your posterior chain – your back, hamstrings and calves. Focus there, and on your quads and core. If you're a rugby player, there's a balance to be struck between upper and lower body strength – work on your ability to transfer power through your body. Here the weight goes up, the reps come down and you typically enter what's known as a 'hypertrophy state' or a muscle-building phase. If you're after functional fitness, like a farmer might be, you can carry on the same movements from the previous phase, but increase your weight and lower your reps. For cardio workouts, start spiking your heart rate and using more of your anaerobic energy system. Think of adding in longer sprint sessions – for example, one to three minutes at a 70 to 80 per cent effort, with the same time at an easy jog/walk to recover; or longer, slower hill climbs to push your heart rate higher, let it recover, and go a bit higher again.

**Here's a sample sprint session:**
Start with a ten-minute warm-up jog at an easy pace. Then do four to six sets of three minutes running at a 70 to 80 per cent effort, with three minutes' rest between each run. Alternatively, do three to five sets of two minutes running up an incline at 70 to 80 per cent effort. Walk downhill to recover. Then warm down with ten minutes' easy jogging.

Understanding the functionality of your house is more important than how it looks on the outside. The exception is a body builder, where it's all about looks; but otherwise, whether you're an athlete or just trying to lose weight – focus on function and performance, and not whether you like what you see in the mirror. Building muscle upon muscle doesn't necessarily carry over into performing better in real life.

With the right focus, the look of your body – your house – simply becomes a byproduct of your hard work towards performance, not the goal itself. There's no point in having a beautiful house where the cupboard doors jam or the hot water doesn't work.

As a farmer, the test is whether you feel good and perform better on the farm, and feel less fatigued. Often you lose weight, gain muscle and look a bit better after following a good training plan, but that's a bonus – it's not the focus. It's how good you feel in day-to-day life – if you've performed better on the rugby field, or on the farm, and don't feel drained after a day running around after the kids.

The next phase is specific. It's about what colour you paint the walls, and the fittings you want in the bathroom. It's a phase geared to your specific athletic pursuit. To get to maximum strength using the extra muscle fibres you've built in the first two stages. They are now being tested to make sure your brain knows how to use them, so they recruit as much muscle as possible to do the work. When lifting weights, cut your reps down to four to eight, but go as heavy as possible, so you're performing at 85 to 95 per cent of your maximum.

I'm training for endurance running these days, so I focus on deadlifts and squats to build my posterior chain muscles (essentially the back of your body, from the calves up) plus my quadriceps. On the cardio side, this stage introduces medium-length interval training, such as 200m to 800m repetitions at pace, and some short, sharp hill reps.

It's a good idea to start your strength training sessions with the biggest movements first, before you start to fatigue.

The more repetitive your training sessions, the more progress you'll see. Try to find that balance between repetition, and adding in something different to keep some variety and excitement in your training. I'll often super-set (do two exercises one after the other) a max-strength movement with a core exercise, or a rehab movement while I rest in between sets to keep me interested.

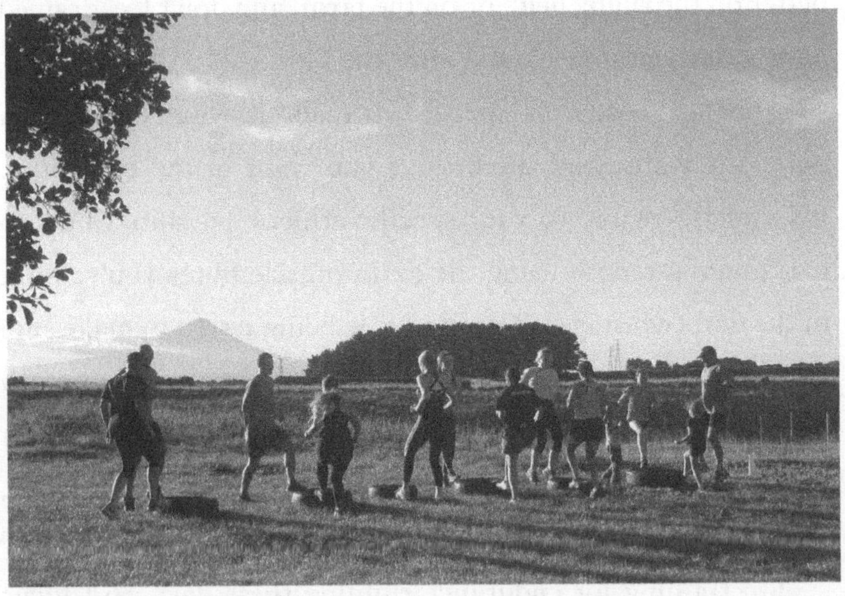

*Farm Fit on a great summer evening.*

A good protocol here is an E2MOM (Every Two Minutes on the Minute). Start a stopwatch before the first rep, and give yourself two minutes to complete A and B, and rest before starting again.

A) Deadlift: 4–8 reps

B) Crunches: max reps

A) Squats 4–8 Reps

B) Superman core holds, max reps. (Lie on your front, arms outstretched above your head, feet slightly apart, and bracing your core and back. Lift all four limbs straight up off the ground and as high as possible. Hold for three seconds, thenlower.)

A) Pull-ups 4–8 reps

B) Russian twists, max reps. (Lie on your back, bending your knees at 90 degrees, so your heels are on the ground. Raise your torso and shoulders off the ground to 90 degree hip flexion, so that you're balancing on your bottom. Then outstretch your arms from your sternum and clasp your hands together and, keeping your eyes and chest in line with your hands, rotate your hands and torso to the left, and then all the way over to the right side of your body. Your hands will make a large arc in front of your body. To progress, lift your heels off the ground and/or hold a weight in your hands.)

A) Bench Press 4–8 Reps

B) One-sided farmers carry, 40m each side

Do this for 3–5 sets.

The final phase is completing the finishing touches on your house so you can move in. For power, you take all that strength you've built in those new muscle fibres and teach them to contract as fast as possible. You can apply plyometric training at this stage: jumping, skipping and bounding. Start using lighter loads, but with maximum force applied and, for cardio, start doing intense ten-second sprints at maximum effort. This will bring your fitness to a peak for a specific event.

You can cycle through all four phases several times in a year; but each time you return to the start, hopefully you are able to lift heavier weights and run faster than the previous time.

Much of what I've shown here is generic, but that's because I believe in functional fitness programmes that can be used by anyone to feel fitter and healthier.

At FarmFit, we have to cater to a huge range of abilities – about half of our regulars are not really habitual exercisers. Perhaps another quarter would be classed as dabblers, and the remainder either play a sport or have a pursuit such as running, cycling or hiking.

Push and pull exercises are central to what we do, because they are efficient, simple and replicate real life. A lot of our sessions are inspired by what I've picked up from CrossFit and Strongman events. Fitness can be as simple or as complicated as you want to make it and, being a farmer, I find simple works pretty well for me. I always aim for the best bang for my buck when choosing movements and protocols to follow. I am a big believer that equipment should not be a barrier in getting to where you want to be.

If you're setting up at home, the secret is finding out what type of workout you enjoy. You're more likely to stay with it then. It's important to be able to build in progression, so you get the benefits of increased fitness and muscle.

My favourite piece of homemade kit is the sandbag. There's a lot of real-life carry over with a sandbag: it's an odd-shaped object, and it doesn't matter if you're a farmer, an accountant or a parent, at some stage you're going to have to pick up a calf off the ground, or shift a heavy box of files, or wrestle a toddler in the middle of a tantrum. Making your own sandbag is cheap and easy. Buy a canvas army duffel bag – it costs about forty bucks. Inside I put a plastic meal sack, but you could use a hessian coffee bag, and fill it up with dirt. Pad out any gaps with old rags or towels. Then cable-tie it, and zip up the duffel bag, securing it with strops and duct tape. You can fill it up to a 60kg weight if you want. Bearhug the bag to your chest and do squats; or deadlift it from the ground; or push-press it above your head to work your shoulders; or lunge with it across your shoulders.

Remember our drench containers? You can replicate them at home using a couple of old buckets. Fill them with water – 10L equals 10kg of weight. They will be perfect for performing the farmer's carry – where you hold the containers straight down by your sides and walk forwards. You can also replicate most of the sandbag exercises.

A tyre is also something you can pick up cheaply, or for nothing. You can box-jump on and off tyres; tyre flips are a great exercise; and whacking a tyre with a sledgehammer replicates the same movement as a woodchop, which is a great full-body exercise.

And finally, get yourself to Mitre Ten and spend 20 bucks on a fence post. You can carry a fencepost as you would carry a calf – it's called a Zercher carry. Hold your arms out in front of you at a 90-degree angle, and rest the post in the crooks of your elbows. A regular fence post might weigh 5kg and a strainer post 20kg, and you can use a barbell with weights on the end if you really want to load up.

All those exercises are ones that can be quite safely completed by a novice without too much instruction and allows them to carry a heavy weight relative to their strength and fitness without injury.

If you want to measure your own progress while working out at home, use our FarmFit fitness test. All you need to replicate it is about 100 metres of fairly flat ground – your local rugby or soccer field would be perfect.

It starts with 30 burpees, then a 100m run. Then do 30 bodyweight squats, 30 pushups and 30 crunches, with a 100m run between each exercise. Repeat it all again, but this time complete 20 repetitions. Then you do a final set, with 10 reps. The fastest person we've had at FarmFit did it in just over 15 minutes, with the slowest about 29 minutes, and the average about 22 minutes. I devised the test because it covers four basic essential movements that can be completed without any equipment, and includes a cardio element that will really push you.

People love to see how they progress over the course of a season.

If you still need some inspiration, here are a couple of sample classes that proved popular with the crew here in Taranaki:

**Session One:**

Warm-up and dynamic stretches for 10 to 15 minutes. Do 80 reps lifting a container from the ground to your shoulder, stopping every even minute to perform 8 pushups, and stopping every odd minute to perform 4 tricep dips. Continue until you've completed the 80 ground-to-shoulder reps with the container. Rest for 3 to 5 minutes.

AMRAP for 12 minutes. Then 6 deadlifts from a range of 35k to 60kg, a 20m sled pull, 60m jog, then rest 3 to 5 minutes.

Then 5 rounds of 12 sledgehammer blows, 12 Russian twists, 25m farmers' carry (heavy load). Then warm down and stretch.

**Session Two:**

Warm up and dynamic stretching for 10 to 15 minutes. Then a ladder workout. Sandbag shoulder press – start at 10 reps and drop 1 rep per round. 30 metre farmers' carry. Sandbag squat – start at 1 rep, and increase 1 rep per round up to 10 reps. Rest for 3 to 5 minutes.

Then a strength test: 120 push-ups. Every time you have to stop for a rest, complete 10 crunches and 20 bodyweight squats. Rest for 3 to 5 minutes.

Then EMOM for 16 minutes:

1st minute: 40m farmers' carry

2nd minute: 10 tyre flips

3rd minute: 40m Zercher post carry – carrying the post in the crook of your elbows

4th minute: 120m run.

Warm down and stretch.

## TOP PADDOCK TOOL

# Motivation

The most common fitness questions I get asked are about motivation. It's usually: 'How do you stay motivated to keep training?' or 'How do you find the motivation to start?'

The answer is I don't. I've learned that motivation disappears faster than a fart in the wind. It's never there when you really need it, so I don't ever rely on it. Requiring motivation to do what you need to do is a fast track to failure.

What they're really asking about is discipline.

It's discipline that is a hundred times more important. Discipline will get you where you need to go. Discipline goes hand-in-hand with something we've already talked about: being able to rely on yourself, and doing what you said you'd do. Discipline is committing to something, and doing what it takes to do it – when it is needed – not when you feel like doing it.

The other skill I've found that most high achievers possess is the ability to refocus when they get distracted. We never really lose motivation, we just tend to get distracted by things and lose our focus on where we were going, or why it was important to us. That's why it's important to understand your 'why' and be able to bring that to the front of your mind when you don't feel like training or doing what you'd promised.

## Chapter ten

# The Circle of Life

FARMERS ARE MORE FAMILIAR with the circle of life than most. We have no choice but to be confronted by it almost every day. If your meat comes shrink-wrapped on a plastic tray, then you don't really have to think about where it came from, and that disconnect for many urban people has only grown. A couple of generations ago I suspect most city-dwellers would have known someone who worked on a farm, and had a connection and understanding of how their food went from pasture to plate. I feel that's no longer the case, and many don't understand that it's possible to both love animals and understand that they have a purpose – and part of it is to feed other things – whether that's us, or lions. It's the food chain.

I've made a point of allowing my kids to experience the realities of life early on. They know about life and death. They've seen calves born and they've also seen dead animals on the farm. They know that we eat some of the cows. I don't try to hide them from it – I don't think that would protect them, it would just create problems for them later in life.

Anyway, I'm not insulated from death, and I'd argue that anyone in the rural sector understands it. But I'm not sure any of that was particularly useful when it came to the most emotionally excruciating experience of my life, one of the harshest examples of nature's indifference towards us I've ever seen.

Lisa Tamati has competed in some of the world's toughest races, such as the Death Valley Ultramarathon and the Marathon des Sables, a multi-stage race run over six days across the Sahara Desert. She's run so hard she's hallucinated seeing penguins in dinner jackets mid-race.

I vaguely knew who Lisa was because she was a New Plymouth local, and I'd seen her adventures and achievements extensively reported. Once Nicole and I began to get into running, the Facebook and YouTube algorithms began serving up her training videos on a regular basis, and I discovered she had a website where she offered coaching to runners. Nicole signed up for her basic training plan, and we joined her Facebook group and began learning from her. She was inspiring, motivating and deeply knowledgeable.

And then, in the spring of 2018, we saw a video Lisa posted to Facebook where she talked about how she was unable to have children, mainly because of the punishment her body had taken from years of ultra-distance running. She was looking for a surrogate mother to carry a baby for her and husband Haisley.

Half-jokingly, I said to Nicole: 'You're really fertile, you could do that,' and she turned around and said: 'Yes, I could.' I think Nicole was searching for a new sense of purpose in life. She'd spent the last few years raising kids and putting up with my rubbish as a struggling farmer. There's nothing easy about being married to a farmer, and I think she may have been struggling with her sense of identity, and her place outside of being a wife and mother. We both thought it would be an awesome thing to help someone else have a baby.

Three days later, Lisa and her mum, Isobel, were at our kitchen table, talking to us. We spoke for a couple of hours, just to get to know each other. Then Nicole and I talked it over for the next few weeks.

I was naive to what surrogacy involved. In this case, they wanted to use Nicole's egg and Haisley's sperm, and for Nicole to carry the baby. That was something of a surprise: I'd imagined Lisa's eggs would still be viable and Nicole would simply carry the embryo for them.

That was a bigger step for me, accepting that my wife would be pregnant to another man and she would have a baby with someone else, who would then live in another family. I really struggled with that for a while. It was a strange feeling.

But in the end, I realised it was up to Nicole to decide to go ahead if she wanted, and that my pride shouldn't get in the way. If she was comfortable with the consequences that her DNA wouldn't be living with her, and if she was happy, I was happy.

The implantation worked at the first attempt. About three months into the pregnancy, we began telling other people. I remember sitting around the table at Christmas explaining it to my family: 'I've got something I have to tell you guys. Nicole's pregnant again.'

They started congratulating us. 'No, no. It's not mine.' Silence. It was good prank to play at the time. Our family took it well, but a few of the people we told clearly thought what we were doing was quite strange.

Nicole and Lisa were both very happy, and I was happy because it felt like the ultimate gift to give someone. It also increased my respect for Nicole – that she could be so selfless – I've often told her she's got an elephant-sized heart in a pocket-sized body.

We got to know each other over the next few months. Lisa helped us a lot with our running, and she provided the final push for me to start FarmFit after I confided to her that I'd dreamed of opening a boxing gym, but didn't feel like I had the knowledge, courage or ideas to take the plunge. She told me to just do it.

**When we have an idea to start something, we often aim for perfection. We research, we ponder and we wait for the stars to align before we start. They never do. There is no perfect time to start – except for right now.**

**Figure out the challenges and pick up the knowledge you need as you go along. Just start – aim for quantity over quality in the beginning. The quality will come with time.**

FarmFit kicked off, and it felt that Nicole and I were both embarking on journeys that gave us both a sense of purpose, and of giving back. It was a good time for us, I think.

When we went to the initial baby scans, I got a real sense of how much this meant to Lisa and Haisley.

They had been trying for some years to have a child together, and they had reluctantly accepted it was unlikely to happen. Now it looked like it might just work out for them.

I remember the 18-week scan was delayed because the clinic was fully booked, so it was about a month late. I couldn't go, because I had to milk, so Nicole went with our two children, and met Lisa and Haisley in New Plymouth. They had the scan, everything seemed fine, and she set off home. About 40 minutes later I got a call from her – she would have been halfway home – to say she was going back because the obstetrician had asked her to return urgently.

I jumped in my car to follow her. When we arrived, there was a midwife, and a specialist doctor in the room. The midwife looked visibly upset, and told me and Nicole quietly that it was not going to be good news. They sat us down, and the doctor told us there was a quite severe problem with the baby. It had spina bifida, a birth defect in which a developing baby's spinal cord fails to develop properly. I didn't really know the implications but Nicole, as a qualified nurse, did and Lisa knew too because she understood the body so well.

There were a lot of tears and disbelief. I felt that Nicole was giving such a great gift, and mother nature had just come in and delivered something terrible. It felt dreadfully unfair that doing such a good thing would bring such a dreadful outcome.

Just under a fortnight later, Joseph was delivered early, at just 24 weeks. There was no expectation that he would survive the birth, but he did. He only lived for two hours, but it was an incredibly precious time.

The day he was born was the most horrible experience I've ever been through. We all spent some time holding and cuddling Joseph – in particular Lisa, Nicole and Haisley – showing him all the love in the world, It was painful to go through, but, at the same time, quite beautiful. I've never been in a room with so much love in it, because you had two couples who were obviously very attached to this baby, and had been through a lot to get to this point. I vividly remember this feeling of a really powerful love.

I have so much respect for how Nicole handled it. She was incredibly strong, and I remember thinking what an amazing woman she was to go through this. To see her love for this child as well was difficult, but beautiful at the same time.

Lisa's parents, Cyril and Isobel, were there. Nicole's mum and dad were there. Everyone spent time with Joseph until he passed away.

It was a very difficult experience to process. I know Nicole really struggled for a long time afterwards with guilt because, even though she was essentially giving a gift, she felt like she'd failed to deliver. It was tough to see her go through it.

It was a crushing blow. Right when we thought life was going really well, we got a left hook that no one saw coming. In one way, it brought us closer together, but in another, it opened up a gulf between us.

I think it was hard for Nicole because I was having success with the farm and with FarmFit, and she had tried to do something to give back and do good for the world, but it left her feeling as if she had failed. I think she carried that feeling of guilt for a long time. I know people would say it wasn't her fault – she was just trying to help – but you can't help how you process your feelings, can you? I didn't know what to say to help. And I felt my success was contributing to how she felt, and that made me feel guilty. I felt like I wasn't entitled to that success, because she was doing a much greater thing than me.

Nicole is very stoic, so I don't think she really showed outwardly how much it was affecting her. But I know it did.

To me, it was a reminder that life is unfair. It doesn't care whether you're doing good or bad.

But I took from that experience how beautiful love was, because that was the overwhelming feeling I got on that day. I try not to look at it as tragic, but beautiful. It's a weird way to frame it, I know. But in that room was a feeling of unbridled love – a type of love I'd never experienced before.

There were some brief conversations about trying again, but it was just too painful, and there was the risk of it happening again. I'm not sure any of us could have handled it again emotionally. At that stage, I think Nicole just wanted to recover, but if she had to, I knew she would do it again – that's the kind of person she is.

I know it was very painful for Lisa and Haisley; it profoundly affected Lisa. It's probably the only thing she felt she had failed at – ever – because if you know her story, she's a conqueror. It was potentially her last shot at being a mother.

I saw all this play out from a step back. Even though I was quite connected to all of them and loved all of them, I was a little less connected to Joseph, and I knew that as much as it was sad for me, it wasn't a patch on what Lisa, Haisley and Nicole were feeling.

We still catch up. We will always feel a part of each other's families, and when we do see each other, Lisa and Haisley feel like a brother and sister to me. Their whole family treats us the same way. They are such good people. We will always have that connection. We found out there was a distant connection – Nicole and Lisa are related through Nicole's grandmother.

There was another link, through Lisa's father, Cyril. About six months before Cyril died, he gave me two of his guns: a .22 and a shotgun. He was an excellent artist, and he painted us a picture when Joseph died. It was a beautiful coastal Taranaki sunset with a view over the ocean. Somehow, in that artwork, he conveyed the beauty and the sadness of what had happened.

Cyril had played rugby for Whanganui and, towards the end of his career, had played club rugby for Bell Block, and it turned out he had actually played rugby with my dad. Dad had just made it into the senior side from high school, and Cyril was still playing in his early forties.

Nicole offered to help Lisa because we had decided our family was complete. But, a year and a half later, we had our third child, Dempsey. To this day, neither Nicole nor I can understand how she became pregnant with Dempsey. We've come to see her arrival as something that was just meant to be – a gift we didn't know we needed until she arrived. When Dempsey was born, we both had the same feeling; it felt right, and our little family felt complete.

### TOP PADDOCK TOOL

## Gratitude and Silver Linings

Let me be straight: there was no silver lining to the passing of Joseph. Nothing ever makes up for that type of loss. But we all have to find some sort of meaning in times of great pain, to help us get through. We needed a way to remember Joseph, and to honour his short life.

It created a unique relationship between the four of us, and I think I felt it first because I was a step removed from it. I remember that love in the room, and I believe each of us, in our own time, learned to love and cherish that love. I felt privileged to have been able to witness it, and I was able to take away that one positive – the memory of bearing witness to so much love in one room, among so much pain and sadness.

When you go out in the storm, you're bound to get wet. At this time in my life, I was putting myself out there with FarmFit, but Nicole had put herself out there to a much greater degree – in a way not many people do – because hers was a gift that you cannot put a price on. When you do something so big and so selfless, you expect it to turn out well. We all felt it was meant to be because it was such a beautiful thing to do. It was a harsh reminder that sometimes the universe doesn't care.

But, while life can be uncaring, you can choose the filter you see it through.

Gratitude is a really important word here. I had begun to practise gratitude a few years before Joseph's short life. Most people see gratitude as sitting down at the end of the day and scribbling down three things you feel grateful for – a roof over your head, a meal in your stomach, and the sun shining. That's fine, but you can get stuck for things to write and end up continually writing down how you're happy to have a home and not be outside sleeping in a tent.

So I've since learned that the most powerful form of gratitude is remembering a time when you either received or witnessed gratitude, and recalling that story and the emotions you felt at the time. I choose to remember when Nicole did something beautiful for someone else, and seeing those people receive it. Now I can sit down and play that story in my mind, and the feelings associated with it. That's my ultimate gratitude story – bearing witness to Lisa and Haisley's emotions and reactions, and how much it meant to them.

When I tap into that memory, I feel privileged to have been a witness to it. I feel some of that gratitude myself, for being allowed to be part of that journey. I feel satisfaction from seeing someone do something so selfless. And most of all, I feel love. I only have positive emotions when I recall that memory.

It's as simple as remembering that special moment and turning it into a story you can tell yourself. It helps to write it down the first time, while paying attention to the feelings you've experienced and witnessed. Over time, it may become as simple as writing down a few words that can trigger the memory and, at that stage, you may find that you can re-tell it to yourself anytime and anywhere. That's why having a gratitude journal, notebook – or even a notes list in your phone – is such a good idea. You can revisit those moments and those feelings whenever you need to.

So finding a time in your life that you witnessed or felt gratitude like that – that's like a gratitude journal on steroids.

## Chapter eleven

# Adapting and Overcoming

THE WORST THING ABOUT DAIRY FARMING? Let me paint you a picture. It's a summer Saturday morning. I've milked the cows, done whatever needed to be done around the farm, and I'm home at 8.30am. Time for a family day out to the beach. But, by the time we grab a feed, bundle the supplies and the kids into the car, and make the long drive, it's nearly 10.30am.

By 1pm it's time to pack up, because at 1.30pm I need to be in the car heading home – I've got to milk those cows again. Afternoon milkings in the summer are possibly the least favourite task for any farmer. I'm yet to meet anyone who enjoys milking in the heat of the afternoon. We don't like it, and the cows don't like it much either – they feel the heat more than we do.

My wife hates it, the kids hate it, I hate it – because no matter how good a time we're having, I still have to go home to those cows. I go back out to work, and my family sits in the house feeling ripped off that their day at the beach only lasted two or three hours.

Aside from the time getting my cows into an energy surplus by 16-hour milking, I'd always been a 'milk twice-a-day, all-year-round' farmer. I'd heard there were some farmers who milked just once a day, and I'd believed the collective wisdom that this approach was just laziness, and a desire for an easy life – perhaps because they were financially secure and didn't really need the income. I look back now and think that attitude was just jealousy – but I had bought into it.

I began to think about the issues we had in the industry – burnout, depression and stress – and how there had to be a better way.

Flipping the pages of a dairying magazine I came across an article that grabbed my attention. It was about a new milking regime where farmers milked 10 times a week instead of 14: twice a day on Monday, Wednesday and Friday; and once a day Tuesday, Thursday, Saturday and Sunday.

Suddenly I saw the prospect of much more freedom on a weekend, family time no longer being such a manic rush, and maybe even enjoying a sleep-in a few days a week.

I'd always considered myself progressive, always willing to embrace new technology and ideas in pursuit of being the best farmer I could. I was familiar with experimenting, but this was something new to me – an idea that was progressive as well as allowing some work–life balance.

16-hour milking meant every second day was the same, regardless of where it fell in the week. One day I'd milk early morning and late night, the next I'd milk mid-morning. But staff struggled with it and it became a pain in the arse. Those late-night milkings mess with the body clock, and milking late morning tends to waste the day, with not much being achieved before or after milking. I'd done it when I had to, but I wasn't a massive fan of how it worked.

But with 10-in-7, I'd follow a far more relaxed 16-hour pattern on weekdays, and on the weekend, I milked once on Saturday morning, once on Sunday morning, and repeat. It was one less milking per week, and a much more family-friendly pattern.

The article talked about a farm consultant in the South Island, Brent Boyce, who had some clients trialling the 10-in-7 technique and while the gaps between milkings were bigger, he'd collected data to suggest the cows were maintaining the same volume of milk production.

This immediately struck me as something I would be willing to have a go at. I thought of myself as someone who was ready to test out new innovations, and this one really piqued my interest.

A few weeks after I read the article, I discussed it with some farming friends. They tried it and reported back that they were happy with how it worked. That gave me the confidence to trial it as well.

**The Seven P's: Proper Prior Preparation Prevents P*ss-Poor Performance.**

**An old one but a good one, I reckon, and a valuable quote to remember for any endeavour in life. Don't think for a second I just turned up to milk one day and decided to implement 10-in-7. I researched it, sought out as much information as possible, talked to others about their experiences trialling it, and then formulated a plan to give it every chance of being successful. Success doesn't often come by chance.**

I discovered there was almost no production loss, and we were milking four fewer times per week. That was 12 hours away from the cowshed, the opportunity to be finished by lunchtime on weekends, to have the afternoon and evening free to spend with the family without having to rush home.

Why were we milking twice a day, seven days a week, when we could do it ten times a week for very little loss?

It wasn't just time I was saving. If I had to get a relief milker in, it meant fewer milkings to pay them for. We used less shed powder, acid and teat spray. The cows loved it, which made milking more enjoyable. I've used the system for three successive seasons now.

Lots of people ask me questions about how it works. Inevitably, the first one is always about how much production I lose. That's understandable, because it's a big component of your profitability. If there's less milk out, there's less money in.

There was an initial drop in production during the first week of the change, but the following week, once the cows settled into their new milking times, production went right back up to what they were delivering on the twice-a-day milking regime.

Think of the long-term effects – like increased staff enjoyment, reduced worker burnout, less stress, less heat stress on the cows (because of that afternoon milking you're avoiding) – and the equation balances up. If you've got people in the cowshed that aren't enjoying it, or struggling to deal with the afternoon heat and accompanying fly problem, they probably aren't doing a top notch job either, and that can end up costing you as well.

When the industry has a severe problem attracting and retaining staff, and keeping them happy, and a bunch of farmers stuck in a cowshed who don't really want to be there, we should try anything new that offers the chance of bringing a better work–life balance; or giving us the opportunity to be out doing more of the higher-skilled tasks; or helping to improve our workforce's skills.

The first year I used the system I switched to 10-in-7 in January, and ran the system for six weeks until COVID-19 first popped up, and the lockdown announcement was made.

Nicole was working two days a week, but, because of the pandemic, was asked to increase that to four days a week. It seemed that as well as panic-buying toilet paper, the general population was also rushing to the doctor. She was an essential worker, as was I, so we could have enrolled the children in daycare, but we discovered they would be the only ones there, and that didn't sound like much fun for them. It became clear I was going to have to spend a lot more time looking after the kids – so I went one step further with the milking revolution, and went to once-a-day milking. I figured if I was ever going to attempt it, this was the perfect time.

In previous years, I'd had the problem of cows coming to the end of the season underweight and having to be fattened up.

I thought that in those final weeks of the season, only being milked once a day would allow the cows to put on some weight: I could keep milking them later into the year but they would be in really good condition when it came time to dry them off.

So on day one of the first New Zealand COVID-19 lockdown on March 25, 2020, I went to milking the cows once a day. It felt liberating. And having the kids out on the farm with me was an absolute blast. I made a point of turning the farm into their classroom, and it made me feel so content seeing their interest in how it all came together to produce food for thousands of people every single day.

In March, April and May, I hit record production for those months: so I got more milk from milking once a day than I had from doing it twice a day. That year, I milked into the month of June for the first time ever, and didn't dry the cows off until June 10. It turned out to be a record season overall for the farm.

The cows dried off in great condition, setting us up for another good season the following year.

Why then, had I been slaving away in the afternoons every March, April and May to get less milk?

It was a game-changer. I'd held these erroneous beliefs – that were actually other people's beliefs – but I had tested them, and found them to be wrong. My whole mindset around milking changed, and my eyes were opened to new possibilities.

People had told me 10-in-7 wouldn't work, that I would lose too much production, that the cows could not handle switching between one milking on a weekend and two on a weekday and would be unsettled. And I thought, to myself that we wouldn't know that until we tried it and, if it failed, I would at least have learned something from the experience.

The next season, I pushed it even further. I started the year milking twice a day through spring, and mating when the cows were at peak production, but I switched even earlier to 10-in-7 on December 23, when the cows were still producing a good volume of milk, despite the prevailing theory that the more milk they are making, the bigger the drop when the regime changes.

I was nervous and worried the loss would be dramatic. The cows had been producing a daily average of 1.87kg of milk solids each at twice a day. That figure dropped, and then a week later it came back up – to exactly 1.87kg. There was the proof. It was clear as day that the cows could handle it. The equation was simple: four fewer milkings, for the same amount of milk. I'd be foolish not to do it.

**You can't truly understand the resilience of something until you test it. We forget that all animals have a resilience and adaptability that's far superior to ours. Like our ancestors, their resilience is defined by the will to survive.**

When I think about it, the cows' resilience and adaptability to change isn't that surprising. Through many of the conversations I've had on this topic, it's our closed minds and the old attachments we hang on to that halt progress.

There's so much change and challenge occuring in agriculture right now – new requirements, red tape and ever-changing standards – and there's a heap more coming in the near future. One of the biggest pressures on landowners now is conforming, changing and adapting to new expectations, and it is often dictated by people with little to no understanding of the realities of farming. A lot of it needs to happen. But change also needs to be backed with science and logic, rather than point-scoring and emotions. It's in these times I'm reminded of a quote by Floyd Mayweather, one of the greatest boxers of all time: 'I'm a winner because I adjust to my environment. I haven't lost – not because of my skills – but because whatever the other guy brings, my desire to win requires me to adapt and adjust to overcome anything. Whoever does that the best in their chosen field always wins.'

**It's human nature to be resistant to change. We all do it to some degree. But winners always adapt. It's no different in my industry: to survive and be successful in the future we must take some leaps of faith and find out what we are truly capable of.**

At the end of March, I changed again to once-a-day milking, and kept milking right through until June 5 again. I had produced far more milk than I had in any previous year. It capped off another really successful season, and I found myself loving farming again.

A lot of what I had envisioned and planned for in the midst of a fairly disastrous time was finally coming together. I had been desperate to solve the problems I was experiencing, and eager to find a balance between working hard, enjoying my work, and being present in my family's life. It finally felt like I was making that equation add up, and it gave me a real sense of relief and accomplishment after years of struggle.

**Hard work works. Manifestation is important: if you have a vision, and an understanding of how you see things eventuating, nothing will happen without doing the work required.**

Another innovation was one of the best investments I ever made – a bit of kit called a Batt-Latch – a computer that runs on a solar panel. It acts as a clock and timer, and opens the gate at the right time for the cows to walk themselves to the cowshed. Instead of driving to the paddock, opening the gate, watching them walk out, closing the paddock and spending 15 to 40 minutes on a motorbike following the cows to the shed, I could be at home and meet them at the shed as the first cows walk into the yard. That saves me half an hour a day, and a whole lot of petrol and boredom idling on my motorbike at 2km an hour, watching cows walking. The cows probably prefer it too, because they can walk at their own speed and are less likely to get lame from being hurried to the shed.

At 2.30pm, I don't have to stop what I am doing and rush to the cowshed. I can spend another 20 minutes on whatever I'm working on. Even better, I pay myself to be with my family.

Let me explain: as a workaholic, I set a price on everything on the farm. There's the mundane, boring jobs like following behind the cow. That's a $20-an-hour job – something anyone could do.

At the other end of the scale are the $100-an-hour jobs: soil testing, pasture management, feed calculations, seasonal planning, doing the accounting – these are highly-skilled, high-level jobs. Putting a price on my time on farm makes me more time-efficient and gives me a greater understanding of my work.

I would always justify being out on the farm instead of being at home because, if I had grass to cut to turn into silage, I could do it myself for free rather than pay a contractor $150 an hour to drive a mower. My labour was effectively free, so I 'saved' that money. That's the mentality a lot of farmers have: they think, 'Oh, f**k that. That's a big bill. It's eight hours' work, but I can do it for free.'

But the reality is that I've got to put a price on my time and a price on running my tractor. Now that I value my time I have to justify being out on the farm. The next question is: 'What am I worth to my family?' So I began paying myself money to be at home, and spending time with the family. And I valued that at $150 an hour because, really, it's priceless.

It allowed me to re-frame my internal debate, so I didn't feel guilty about being at home playing with my kids when there were jobs waiting for me outside. It gave me peace.

The transactions were all mental, of course: no money really changed hands. I would price up a day out with the family on the beach, and I would price up the cost of the contractor. And it would break-even, so I wasn't losing anything. It was a mind trick, but it worked; it made my family happier, and it made me happier. In the past three years, I've spent way more time with them, and now I wouldn't have it any other way.

Early in my career, I put all the value on where I was on the ladder – everything was considered through the filter of whether it got me closer to farm ownership.

But that was someone else's measurement of success, not my own.

I thought I wanted to achieve farm ownership. But what I really wanted to achieve was to recreate that magic, that fun, that adventure of my childhood. Was I getting any of that from a relentless pursuit of farm ownership? Not really.

When I considered my purpose, and what success looked like to me, I realised I could achieve it without owning a farm. What was more important – those title deeds, or raising children in a great environment?

I decided I wasn't willing to sacrifice my relationship with my kids to put in the relentless work required to own a farm, or – at least – not by following the traditional pathway to get there.

It was difficult. Early on in that mental journey, I admit I blamed Nicole a little, because I felt her pulling away from the farm life when I was working far too hard. It caused friction, pressure and stress, and I suspect she didn't want to be part of it anymore; after all, she'd never wanted to be a farmer in the first place. At the same time, I thought if she didn't buy into me working 100 hours a week, then I wasn't going to be able to buy a farm. Once again, I began to question why I was farming.

There's obviously some freedom in owning your own land. But I realised it was not a sacrifice I was willing to make – on my family's behalf – to achieve it.

The reality is that to own my own farm, I would need to move to a significantly larger farm of 600 cows or more, take on more debt and more pressure, and/or take on a second farming job. That's not unheard of. Often people stay working their own farm, but then contract another farm and employ a manager to work it. Of course, that means there are times where you're needed in two places at once.

I ran through both scenarios, and I didn't like either of them, because they both took me away from my purpose. I also realised that the earliest I would end up owning a farm was around 45 years of age, and by then my oldest daughter would be ready to leave home, and I would have missed her childhood. Without relying on the capital gains previous generations had enjoyed, would all that sacrifice be worth it?

I haven't given up on that dream – I still have a strong desire to own my own patch of dirt – but I doubt it will be achieved by taking the traditional pathway.

Farm ownership no longer defines my success. It has gone from a 'need' to a 'want'. I can be content with or without it, because it's not my sole purpose in life, as it once was. There are a thousand ways to make enough equity to get into land, and it's been my loss – and that of many others – that we've all been blindly following only one of those pathways, simply because that's what farmers have done for the last few generations.

It's a brave step to throw away other people's ideals of success, and be honest enough to decide that's no longer your measurement of success. Go and ask 100 farmers at the bottom end of the ladder. Every single one would tell you their goal is to own their own farm, but in truth, the majority will not be willing to make the massive sacrifices to get there.

It has taken a few years for me to accept that reality. In the years of the low payouts, the reality had begun to dawn, and I began to understand my purpose.

Purpose, to me, is like an intimate relationship. When you first get together, and it's all going well, you're as close as an index finger and a thumb – you feel connected and it's a strong bond. As the years go by, you get challenges and differences, and the bond can stretch and feel a little distant. The bond ebbs and flows at different times. It's the same with your purpose: when it feels like it is ebbing away, you start to question why you're still doing this thing. Reconnecting with my purpose was like reigniting a relationship. I now run all my decisions through the filter of that purpose and ask myself: 'Does this fit?'

**Struggling with your passion or wondering why you're doing what you're doing? Then go back to why you started in the first place, ask yourself the hard questions. Do you still hold the same values, beliefs and dreams as you did then? There's a reason why you started in the first place. Does that reason still resonate with you?**

It was a journey to bring my purpose back, and understand why I was there and what I was doing.

FarmFit has helped me significantly with that journey, and particularly the people I've met as a result. I have written a lot about the negativity I have seen around farming, and the impact that has had on my mental health.

But FarmFit's growing social media presence had an unintended, but very welcome, consequence of introducing me to a lot of new people who were positive about farming, and life in general. It was a group of people who, like me, believed in doing good and helping others, and had this upbeat, positive attitude to the industry and to life itself. They exuded energy and that, in turn, gave me a renewed energy for life.

The first time I experienced that feeling was about ten months into FarmFit's existence. I had about 300 followers at the time, and reaching 500 was my goal. I filmed a short video sitting on my tractor talking about a quote I'd heard on a podcast: 'Float like a duck and paddle like f**k.'

I thought it was a great analogy for life – we're all trying to look graceful on the surface, like we've got our sh*t together – but underneath the water, we're paddling like mad to keep up with life. After ruminating on it for a while, I stopped the tractor on the way back to the cowshed, and did a quick video about how much this line had resonated with me.

It was a little different to the content I usually shared, so at first I was hesitant to post it. But the next morning, during morning milking, I got a Facebook message from a guy in my running group. It was a screenshot of the New Zealand Farming Facebook page – they'd re-posted my video and his comment was: 'Kane, you're famous!'

The New Zealand Farming page has 220,000 Facebook followers, and another 60,000 on Instagram. When they shared my video it had thousands of likes, thousands of shares, and hundreds of comments. I was stunned.

I didn't have a FarmFit Facebook page, just a personal one, but when I opened up the FarmFit Instagram account, it had gained a thousand followers overnight. It was overwhelming, and I even became a little anxious – I'd mustered up the courage to speak to a couple of hundred people, but now there were thousands, and it kept growing. I put my phone away and got on with the day – until I got a message from a bloke named Tangaroa Walker.

Tangaroa is a Southland dairy farmer whose online education hub, Farm 4 Life, has a huge following: 150,000 on Facebook alone. He'd been an influence early on for FarmFit – seeing his work teaching people and acting as a positive role model. I thought, 'Here is this smart guy, in the trenches, delivering great messages. But he shouldn't have to do it all on his own.' The real power for change comes from everyday people like me – the farmer down the road – and the next one along. We all need to create a more positive, open and honest mindset.

**Ever wonder why your mates who are struggling don't reach out and talk about their battles? It's probably because you haven't either. People will talk when they feel confident they won't be judged – they will reach out to people they feel safe around. If we want people who are struggling to speak up, the responsibility falls on every single person to make vulnerability feel as normal as breathing. People who are struggling will talk to people that talk about their struggles.**

Tangaroa asked me to call him when I was free. I remember messaging him back saying I was a bit busy and would call him another day. I was, to be honest, a bit overwhelmed. Two seconds later my phone rang. I answered.

'Chur brother, Tangaroa here. Just seen your video, bro! Bloody good to see another handsome fella putting his mug out there for everyone to see.'

We had a laugh and a yarn about who I was, and who he was, and I was quite excited that he'd taken the time out to talk to me, because I felt he was quite a big deal. I also wondered if he was also checking me out to see who the competition was, but he told me he thought what I was doing was great.

**Farming has always had a strange dynamic – the unspoken competition between farmers. It's as if you hide the secrets of your success from your neighbour so they can't copy and enjoy it too. I don't know where it comes from but sh*t – we are all in this together, and one farmer's success doesn't detract from anyone else's achievements. We should all actively share more knowledge and help each other succeed. The more farms there are running a profitable, sustainable and enjoyable business model, then ultimately the better off our people, land, animals and country will be.**

Tangaroa and I kept in contact, and a year or so later I interviewed him for the FarmFit page for a show I call 'Cut Loose with Kane-O' – a kind of live podcast where we can interact and be asked questions on the fly by people watching. I reminded him about that first call, and how I felt he might be checking me out and seeing just who I was. He admitted he was – but then he explained that what I hadn't realised was he called me to help himself, because it was lonely doing what he did, and it felt empowering to see me doing the same thing.

'I was ringing you to offload some of my stuff, to make me feel a bit less lonely,' he said.

I do the same thing myself now, because I know it is hard to put yourself out there, and it is lonely at times. I understood him completely. I've got quite a network of positive people like Tangaroa now, and it is a great resource and reassurance, and something I can feed off.

I was invited to Fieldays in Hamilton by NZ Farming founders Duncan Humm and Tyler Fifield to hang out with them for a few days. Along with meeting some awesome farmers and sharing stories, I got to hang out with and get to know Dunc, Tyler, Tangaroa and Laura Koot from farmskills workshop Real Country. They all exude positivity and an infectious energy, and I've learned a lot from all of them. They, and others, are helping build a positive energy for agriculture and over the last few years having access to their energy has helped feed mine.

That's been tremendously helpful for me, because the last year has been one of huge change.

**You become your environment. Who you spend time with, who you listen to, and who you watch ultimately dictates what you think about and what you do. What you do is what you become.**

## TOP PADDOCK TOOL

# Visions, Goals and Actions

Ask people about where they want to go in life and, invariably, they will write down a list of goals.

That was certainly the case in the dairy industry, where it was hammered into every aspiring young farmer that they had to hit specific intermediate goals before they got to the big one: owning their own farm. That was the end result, and it was assumed that was why everyone was farming.

What I found over the more difficult years of my career was that those goals, and the way I was measuring success, no longer lined up with each other. While I'd had those goals, I never felt able to picture what my life would be like in ten years' time.

When I realised that everything didn't quite line up, and I was using the industry's or other people's measure of success, I worked on substituting those fixed long-term goals with a vision. It's much more powerful to create the vision first, then work backwards from that, so you know your goals will align.

If you write down your goals, it can feel incredibly hard to change them – even if you've had children or found a new passion, or life has shifted to make those goals no longer achievable or desirable. It can be really hard to cross them all out and write in new ones without feeling like a failure.

But these fixed long-term goals were preventing me from adapting to life. The goals I had when I began farming eight years earlier, with no kids and a very different farm environment to the one I find myself in now, were no longer so appropriate. The farm ownership pathway is no longer the same – it has become much harder to secure land ownership by the traditional method – and I had to think about whether it was still what I really wanted out of farming.

The exercise I undertook – and which I encourage you to do as well – was to sit down and simply daydream about what I wanted to do in five years, and in ten years' time. What did a good working day look like to me? What am I doing? Who's there? What does my routine look like?

I can see a house up on the crest of a hill. I can see my alarm going off at 6am, and eating breakfast with the kids. I can feel some emotions – principally satisfaction – that this is my ideal day. The vision doesn't mean imagining living in a mansion and never working a day in my life. I haven't won millions on the lottery. It's a realistic and achievable vision of a happy life. I can see the type of work I'm doing, the kind of people I am doing it with, and all the different things it will involve.

I could still be a dairy farmer in that scenario – but probably not milking cows twice a day – which is a realistic view of where I will be in ten years' time.

It made me look at my goals in a very different way. I now only set short- and medium-term goals, and my vision looks after the long term. The vision changes.

Four times a year I sit down and have the daydream, and elements of it change. When I began FarmFit, I realised I had a passion for service to others, so that became a new part of my vision. I can be flexible how that service element will figure in my life, but I know it will be there. When I faced relationship difficulties my vision had to change again. But I didn't have to sit down and rip a page of goals out of my notebook.

I don't look much further ahead now than about six months when goal-setting. I can adjust and adapt to a changing world without feeling like a failure, and without a fixed destination. I'm not working to someone else's measurement of success, but my own vision of how I want my life to look.

A vision is unique to you. You're not living anyone else's definition of success, or by anyone else's measures but your own. You're not in competition with anyone else. People get influenced by the industry they are in to climb the ladder, and we end up with teachers who become head teachers, and realise they've moved away from the part of the job they loved: the classroom.

Actions lead you towards your goals and vision. Your habits are the little things you do every day that help tick off a goal, or lead you closer to fulfilling a vision. Goals without actions are worthless.

One of my goals is to run an ultramarathon, and the action I need to take is to create good habits that support that goal. When I want to go for a run after work, I leave my running shoes and socks at the front door so I almost trip over them when I get home. The habit is not 'going for a run' – the habit is putting out my shoes to trigger me to go running. Likewise, if I know I need to stretch, I leave the foam roller on the couch so I can't sit down and watch television without sitting on it, and that prompts me to get on the floor and roll around for a bit. Studying for a qualification? Leave a book on your pillow or kitchen table. It's a cue to kick the action off. Actions lead towards goals and visions. It's all a chain, and they should all be aligned. The ideal is for as many of your daily actions as possible to feed directly into achieving a goal – and that goal leads you one more step towards fulfilling your vision.

## Chapter twelve

# Embracing Uncertainty

IN THE HEIGHT OF SUMMER, the sun rises here at 5.30am. By then, I've been up for about 90 minutes. As the first rays peek over the horizon, they illuminate the cowshed as I milk the cows, singing along to the Rock Radio's Morning Rumble show. I'm usually a third of the way through, 60 cows done, and 120 or so to go. The cows are chewing on their food, the milking machines are making their rhythmic noise and Roger Farrelly, Andrew Mulligan and Bryce Casey are a bit louder than that. I'm in my gumboots, overalls and apron, and as the sun beats in I'm usually thinking about how peaceful it is, and how lucky I am. I ponder on the day ahead, the jobs I need to do, and the challenges they might pose. But at that moment, I simply try to enjoy the warmth of the sun, the contentment of the cows, and feel a bit of gratitude that I've chosen this path.

The sunset brackets the other end of the day. At 8.30pm I can look up from the paddock at the end of a bootcamp session, or from my deck, and scan the horizon – from the picture-perfect Mt Taranaki some 40km away, to the township of Hawera, to the last rays as the sun dips over the Tasman Sea. It's quite a view.

As I enter my final months farming here, I feel that after all the stress, sweat and tears, I will leave something of myself behind in the place. But I am prepared for fresh challenges and a new view of our mountain.

On the surface, my six-year marriage to Nicole was good and strong but, underneath, even after 12 years together, there had always been issues we had left unresolved.

It led to a brief separation, and, during that time, some honest conversations where we tried to address some of our fundamental issues. But after muddling along for a few more months, it was all over.

It was a horrible conversation – by far the hardest thing I've ever had to do. But it also felt like the right thing to do. The end of our relationship came during what was already a time of great change.

I had told farm owner Brian Williams earlier in the year that, after nine seasons, we would be leaving at the end of the 2022 season. I wanted to find a bigger sharemilking job. There was no opportunity to progress staying where we were, and I was keen to take on new challenges with a larger herd of around 300 to 400 cows. We also wanted to be nearer to Nicole's family in New Plymouth. The location was a compromise to try and make Nicole happier about farm life, but our relationship was not strong enough to handle taking on the complications, and the increased levels of debt that would come with buying a bigger herd.

But ending the relationship also ended the chance – for now – of continuing as a herd-owning sharemilker, and we sold our herd. That was heartbreaking. Transforming the herd over the last nine years has been my proudest achievement in farming to date. You would not recognise them from the scruffy, underperforming bunch that caused me so much stress and worry when I first bought them. It's going to be very hard to say goodbye to them, but I made finding them a good home a higher priority than the sale price.

The break-up was the hardest thing I've ever endured. I played the situation out in my mind before it happened, but I had not anticipated how painful it would truly be. The pain of my three children going to live an hour away, the pain they were in, and the pain Nicole was in, left me buckled over.

Nicole and I separated right at the start of calving. It was the absolute worst time to do it.

I went into the most stressful part of the season while undergoing the most emotionally challenging time I've ever been through. For the first ten days I was in survival mode. I struggled to eat, drink, shower or think. I've never cried so much in my life. I could be sitting at the table eating lunch or out on the farm, and I would unexpectedly break down in tears. I hadn't expected to feel so much pain. I can't even imagine how Nicole felt. I felt pain for her. I felt pain for my kids. I felt pain for me. I'd never experienced grief like this before, but the end of a long relationship is filled with grief. I had lost the family unit I valued so highly, and I realised that family time would never be the same again, and my future was now deeply uncertain.

**Throughout my life I have used training and exercise to help me through hard times. This situation was no different. But I want to make it clear it's not – and never should be – the only tool. You wouldn't go out fencing with just a hammer, would you?**

**It's important to develop many tools and strategies, and learn to use the right one for the right job. I called on every trick and tool I possessed to make it through this time. I even went back through my own Instagram page, and re-watched and re-read my own work to remind myself of everything I knew that might help me to start functioning and looking after myself again.**

What helped me emerge from the pain was an idea I'd had a few months earlier – organising a charity event for I Am Hope, the charity set up by Mike King, which provides mental health care for young people.

I'd spoken briefly to Elle Perriam some months earlier. She'd established the rural mental health charity Will to Live after her own partner, a young farmer, sadly took his own life.

I told Elle that I would be interested in making it a joint fundraiser for her charity as well, and asked her to give me a ring some time to discuss the idea, but I hadn't heard back from her.

In 2020, I had organised a off-road half-marathon where everyone – including myself – ran in gumboots. We raised $7500 for I Am Hope.

Since then, there had been quite a few people complete runs in gumboots – some of them over remarkably long distances. I didn't want to turn the concept into a competition about who could run the furthest, or raise the most; I didn't want that to be the motivation.

I also felt that people were being asked more and more to dip into their own pockets to donate to charities, with so many events and so many dedicated charity days that there was some 'charity fatigue' in the community.

It also seemed to me that the agricultural industry was in a period of strength, with a high milk payout and the rest of the country reeling from the effects of the first wave of the COVID-19 pandemic.

I decided that, instead of organising a run where people were asked to donate to a Give A Little page, we could do something entirely different, with a focus on encouraging rural companies to sponsor the event, and get some positive media attention for themselves.

I came up with the concept of a single day where anyone could get out in their gumboots and log a run on the activity tracking app Strava, and all those individual efforts could be totalled up – with the collective goal of covering the length of New Zealand – about 1600km. Companies could offer a sponsorship fee per kilometre, giving farmers the feeling that, by downing tools, pulling on their boots and going for a 2km trot around their paddocks they were doing something good for themselves – and raising money for charity without dipping into their own pockets.

It felt like a different way of fundraising that motivated people to do something for the cause – and actually think about it – while doing something for themselves.

As part of this concept, I thought about how I could challenge myself, and I decided my goal for this event really had to be running 100km. I've always wanted to run an ultramarathon and while my first thought was to run 50km, I already knew I was capable of completing that distance. I needed the challenge of something really big that made me nervous, and left me with that feeling of uncertainty about whether I could complete it.

I found it incredibly difficult to find the balance between farming, family and training for this event and – to my surprise – to find companies willing to provide sponsorship for these two important charities. Many of the big rural corporates that aren't already supporting national charities were unwilling to help – with the honourable exception of Goldpine – and that got me thinking.

Nearly every company these days seems to have made some gesture in the direction of mental health. I've certainly contributed interviews and articles for businesses wanting to do their bit for raising mental health awareness. But trying to raise funds for the people actually providing services and making a real change for those who are struggling has made me wonder how much of the discussion around mental health is just lip service – a token gesture. It leaves me with the horrible suspicion that some of the rhetoric may not be as genuine as it ought to be. Awareness is no longer the issue – mental health has never been talked about and publicised so much. What's needed now is action.

Just a little over a month after Nicole and I split up, I was sitting on a tractor feeding out to the cows when the phone rang. It was Elle Perriam. I didn't really feel like talking, but I answered. When she asked how I was, I said: 'Well, not great,' and explained what had happened.

She was young when her parents divorced, so she talked me through a child's view of a relationship breakdown, and it was helpful for me to get that perspective. Then she asked about my offer to raise money for her charity so I told her about my plan for the gumboot run. She told me she was about to launch an initiative called Rural Change, which offered free counselling for anyone connected to the agricultural industry, just as I Am Hope provides the same service to children and youth in the same situation.

I'd told her how confused I was and how much pain I was suffering. I felt overwhelmed and was struggling to find a way through these emotions.

Elle asked me how open-minded I was. She told me about a guy she thought would be perfect to help me out. He was a traditional Maori healer. I had never heard of such a thing, so she explained what a Honohono session involved, and how it had helped her. She said it was very different to how a psychologist or counsellor would usually work, which was why I needed to be open-minded.

I thought about it and, although I was incredibly sceptical, I knew I was in a mental state I had to get out of. That meant I was willing to try anything to work through the pain and emotions I had been battling. I booked the next available session with Dion Freeman from Healing Aotearoa. It turned out to be an incredible experience.

Shortly before our lunchtime session, he sent me a link on Zoom, the online meeting platform. He was in the South Island, and I was on my farm in Taranaki, so the whole experience was to be virtual. I was mystified as to how that could possibly work.

But I duly clicked on the link at midday and the man who appeared at the other end introduced himself, and said: 'Kane, for the last half an hour, I've been feeling what you've been feeling.'

I had a wry grin on my face when I replied: 'Oh yeah?'

'This is going to sound really strange,' he said, 'but I've been out for a walk for the last 30 minutes and I've been able to feel your emotional pain in parts of my body.' He spent the next 15 minutes describing the physical pains he had felt in his body, and the significance of each of them. He said how the pain in his hips represented paternal instinct, and how I felt pain about my kids. He went to his heart, and said this was romantic pain, and asked if there was trouble with a partner, or previous partner. He talked about a huge pain in the top of his head, as if there was a block of ice sitting there, and that represented frustration. He said my frustration was through the roof. To me, that represented how I felt about my relationship. He described it perfectly – like my frustrations had got to a point where I couldn't handle them any more.

I was pretty lost for words. I didn't really say anything at all. We'd just been introduced, and in those 20 minutes he explained everything that I was feeling precisely. None of that information was publicly available – I'd dropped off social media and very few people knew I had split from Nicole.

I still remained sceptical. He said he could tell I had a logical brain, and didn't believe him yet. He spent a few minutes explaining what would happen next. 'Just keep an open mind,' he said. 'A lot of people feel the same way as you, but I've done this many times. I'm going to be able to help you – to help relieve some of that pain.'

He told me to lie down somewhere I could be relaxed, and without distractions. He was going to end the conversation, and send me another Zoom link where we could talk again in an hour's time. In the meantime, he said, he was going to be wholly in touch with my body. 'I'm going to go through your body and sort out some of your sh*t that's going on, because I can tell there is a lot there.'

All I had to do was to lie there and picture his face. Any time I felt distracted, or wanted to take control, I had to picture his face again and just let go. 'I know you're going to try and fight it, but just let it go. Let me take over.'

Dion explained some of the sensations I might experience, which took me by surprise and, again, raised my suspicions.

He told me that even though my eyes would be closed, my eyelids might flicker and I would feel the muscles around the eyes twitching. I might hear noises, especially in my stomach. My ears might pop. My joints might click. I might even experience visions.

Remember, I was desperate, and I was willing to try anything. I decided that if it worked, it would be worth it, and if it didn't, well nobody else in the world would ever have to know.

So I lay down on the couch and pictured his face, and by the time my head hit the pillow, my eyelids were flickering. I felt myself trying to hold on to control for probably the next five or ten minutes. I actively had to tell myself to let go. I guess that's probably quite a natural reaction.

I began to get some of the physical sensations he had described: I felt the blood rushing to my head in waves, similar to the feeling you get when you are upside down. The blood would rush up and I felt pressure for about fifteen seconds before it would dissipate, then the next wave would come. Then my tummy began to gurgle. I had my hands resting on my stomach, but I felt as if they were somehow detached from my body and levitating two feet above it.

About half way through the session I started hearing very loud, angry screams, as if I was yelling out. Then, even though my eyes were closed, I began to see outlines of vague shapes – imagine staring at something, then closing your eyes, and seeing the faint remains of that image. The visions began to flick past at increasing speed, and it was coupled with the screaming, the rushing blood, and the continued tummy rumbling. Re-telling this very surreal experience is difficult, because I do not believe in any of this stuff. I am not spiritual. I don't believe in ghosts, clairvoyants or crystal balls.

But I just can't explain it. I can't explain it and I can't explain how he knew some of the things he said. I don't see there's any way he could have found out those details about my life. There's no book he could have read – very few people know my story – and those who do wouldn't know the intimacies that he did. It's opened my mind; I now accept that there are things in this world that defy a logical explanation.

A lot of people will read this and laugh. So what? It

happened, and I am strong enough to handle it if people don't believe me. I have suggested to others that they try it, and to approach it with an open mind. And I admit, if I were listening to myself, I wouldn't believe it. I can try and convince you as you read this, but it's probably something you couldn't accept and believe until you'd experienced it.

Dion told me to set an alarm for an hour after our first call ended. It sounded, and I got up from the couch thinking: 'What the f**k was that?'

I hit the Zoom link and there he was. 'You've got a lot of sh*t going on,' he said. I told him what an intense experience I'd had.

For the next 20 minutes, he told me about my life. He discussed details I had never told anyone. He talked about Nicole and our relationship in highly accurate detail. He talked about our relationships to our parents. He told me I was still trying to make my dad proud of me: 'Every day you go out and work, and you feel like your dad's on your shoulder, and you're trying to prove to him that you can do it.' He told me my dad was proud, and always had been. That was quite a powerful affirmation to hear. I know it's something that would be easy to make up, but it instantly gave me comfort.

The way Dion explained the relationship dynamic between my dad and I, and my wife and I, was spot on.

He also talked to me extensively about the future, and my vision of how I wanted my life to unfold. That was the real clincher for me: he explained it with absolute clarity. I had been working hard for several years trying to understand what I wanted out of life, and where I saw it going. I'd developed a clear vision of how I pictured my future, but I'd never told a soul about how it looked, and yet he nailed it in complete detail.

He asked me about charity and asked, 'Have you got any plans in the future of doing something for charity?'

I was amazed: 'I've just started planning a charity event.'

He said, ' I can see all that in you. I can feel your service to people. I can feel your logic and your problem solving.' Then he said, 'You're capable of way more than you're currently doing.'

I had been experiencing precisely that feeling when I was out on the farm doing basic minimum-wage tasks, and I felt as if my skillset wasn't being properly utilised. Working on a small farm means I do a wide variety of tasks, but also means a lot of menial chores. I came to the conclusion that I was perhaps worth more than spraying weeds.

He touched on trauma I'd had as a child, and how I still held on to it. He even suggested I go and do some boxing or ju-jitsu to release that tension – and then decided it had to be ju-jitsu, because boxing could be a bit too much at my age, and I might end end up hurting myself. I definitely needed some outlet for my fighting spirit and aggression.

He also said I needed a creative outlet; I was a logical person, and a natural problem-solver, but that needed a creative balance. I actually clapped for a moment when he told me that, because I have noticed how good I often feel when recording FarmFit videos – it's energising and testing because I am not a media professional. He also suggested I play guitar – and I told him how, as a teenager, I played a lot of guitar, was in a couple of bands, and found it very helpful. He said it was time to return to it.

And he also told me: 'At this moment in your life, you need to prioritize looking after yourself, because you're not at the moment, and you haven't been.'

For the 40 minutes he spoke to me, there was not one sentence Dion uttered that was incorrect. He seemed to completely understand everything about my life.

He also talked about Nicole, how he could feel her pain, and how immense it was. He believed she would return to me at some stage, as a different woman.

He said my pride got in the way of me being able to move on from certain things in life – particularly our relationship – and I instantly understood what he meant by that. I had to move past that pride to be able to move on. I felt he was describing the first two years of our relationship, which were tough because we were young and fell in love so deeply, and we didn't have the tools to properly communicate and understand each other's perspective. Looking back, I think that inability to communicate clearly caused a lot of damage to the relationship, which we never resolved, and instead just simply ignored. Pride can be a good thing, but it's also a really big obstacle to being vulnerable, being honest and moving on with life.

It was an incredible experience – one I am really grateful for. Immediately after speaking to Dion, I felt a lot of the hurt and guilt – a huge weight – had been lifted from my shoulders.

I still felt the pain and my situation still felt difficult, but I was able to function again. I'd hate to think what state I would be in now without that session, because I probably wouldn't have been able to dig myself out alone. It gave me an insight into myself – and my relationships – that I'd never got anywhere else. I consider that day a huge turning point for me.

**People worry too much about the cost of the shovel when they are using it to dig up gold. I've been there myself – I considered the price of consulting a farm advisor, counsellor or personal trainer too expensive. I didn't think about the extra income they could generate for me, or the costs they might save – not to mention the potential stress, worry and waste of time that could be avoided by using their knowledge to help make me, my family, or my business better. Remember: you are the most important cog in your machine. If you're good – or better than before – everything else will improve too. The investment is worth it.**

In 2021, I began doing some public speaking. I made an inauspicious start at the Hawera A & P Show, where they had a little corner in the show hall with a rotating cast of about 20 speakers, each asked to talk for about 15 minutes. I can admit to you that I was incredibly nervous.

Then I realised I didn't really have an audience – there were maybe two or three people watching me – my job was to try and capture the attention of anyone who wandered past. In hindsight, it was a pretty horrible experience – I figured it could only get better, and I reassured myself that if I had managed to talk to nobody, then I could talk to anybody.

The next gig was talking to the entrants and sponsors of the Taranaki Dairy Industry Awards. I was asked to talk about FarmFit, how it worked, the importance of physical and mental fitness, and the connections I've made since getting on social media.

My biggest gig was the East Coast Farming Expo at Wairoa, where most farming is sheep and beef. They run a Fieldays-type event, with some exhibitors, and a large marquee for meals and seminars. They had an impressive range of speakers and my spot was at lunchtime, called 'Cuppa with Kane-O'. The audience got a sit-down meal and I spoke for an hour.

One thing I've learned about confidence is that if you don't have it, you have to fake it until it feels real.

Before giving a speech, I delved into how people did it. FarmFit bootcamps helped, because that's similar to speaking to an audience – I'm directing, talking, joking and guiding the group through a workout.

I have to have a concept in my head of how I want it to look – I mentally put myself into the audience and watch myself. How do I want to be perceived? How do I act?

I watched a lot of TEDx talks and YouTube videos of public speaking, trying to absorb their confidence.

What does confidence look like? It starts with posture and the way you sound.

Initially, I was acting, and that may sound disingenuous, but it was a way to build up my confidence until it felt real. If I walked into a room with my shoulders down, looking at the floor, it's hard to come back from that. As nervous as I was, I had to fake that confident demeanour until it became a natural confidence.

These events helped keep me in the orbit of some inspirational people who have now become part of my life, including Tangaroa Walker, Elle Perriam and Mike King.

An unintended consequence of FarmFit's success has been to meet and create connections with these people, who are extraordinary in their service to others, and really good for my energy levels.

They've got me excited about the farming industry again, and about the people involved in it.

For a decade, I lived with a ladder of achievements fixed in my head. I've shifted away from that, and now I think more in terms of a vision for my life – a personal picture of how I actually want my life to look each day. That vision is almost like a daydream, which adjusts and flows with life. There are a hundred different pathways to achieving my vision, and I've realised mine doesn't have to include the traditional route of farm ownership. Our pathways don't have to be on a straight line – we should feel free to explore any tangents.

Uncertainty isn't a bad thing. We try to hang on to certainty, because it means safety, but we need to be comfortable enough to accept some uncertainty. You might bet your life savings on the All Blacks beating Fiji every day of the week, but there's still that slender chance it might not happen. There are no guarantees with anything.

Every dairy farmer now faces some uncertainty about how they will be farming in ten years. There's a lot of external pressure to change how we farm. There's also the looming possibility of 'fake' or lab-grown meat, the trends towards vegetarianism and veganism, and increasing government regulation around issues like fresh water, winter cropping, emissions, and the treatment of cows. For example, many farmers in Southland now think they will have to build barns to winter their cows in, which will be a huge expense, and a change to the image of how we farm. Everything is changing fast, and what the industry will look like in a decade is up for debate. In the past ten years, the industry's major players, Dairy NZ and Fonterra, have put out adverts that cast what we do in a very positive light, but we should actually be honest about the mistakes we have made. The industry critics say we haven't owned up to the environmental damage we've caused, and I think they might be right. We should acknowledge that some of our practices 50, 20 or even 10 years ago weren't right, and own up to that. We didn't have the knowledge then that we have now, and we are trying to change and adapt as research and technology allows us. We can't change what was done in the past, only how we approach the future. The industry I began working in 12 years ago was very different to the one I find myself in now. There's a much higher emphasis placed on animal welfare and the environment, and a much better application of technology to drive a better future.

But I have some certainties about the way ahead: I love working with the land. I love the animals. I've got an insatiable appetite to learn and it gives me energy. FarmFit has taken me beyond my comfort zone and I've learned so much from it – I've discovered I enjoy being of service to people. Now I'm fitting those jigsaw pieces together, planning to do some consultancy work, more speaking, developing FarmFit and continuing my love of learning new skills.

I will go contract milking again – where I get a fixed dollar amount for every kilogram of milk solids produced and I'm not at the whim of the milk payout. It's less risk, but also less reward. Some would see that as a step back – I see it as a step to the side to reassess and re-evaluate.

The herd at my new place is 320-strong, which equates to enough cows for me to employ another labourer, and possibly even a part-timer as well. Because the farm has a good rotary cowshed with cup removers, allowing one person to milk the whole herd easily, there will be times of the year where one person could comfortably manage alone. That offers much more opportunity for work–life balance – less time in the shed, more time with the kids, and time to consider other pursuits. But FarmFit will definitely come with me. I will dismantle all the equipment, rebuild it, and introduce myself to a new community.

It will be a different style of dairying. The farm has a herd home, which looks like a giant version of those polythene tunnels for growing vegetables. It's an open-ended barn with a clear, arched roof where the cows can feed, and keep warm when it's wet and cold; they can still go outside when they want to. I'm expecting a wetter and colder climate, and a very different challenge. The owner is also new to it, so it's a fresh opportunity for us both.

The new farm is a 20-minute drive from New Plymouth, much closer to the kids, and right in the bushline of the lower slopes of Mt Taranaki. I will still have a spectacular view of our maunga to wake up to every day, and remind myself just how lucky I am.

## TOP PADDOCK TOOL

# Vulnerability

Nicole's grandfather, Kev, was a tough old bugger. A former dairy farmer and meat worker, he was that type of character who, if he didn't like you, would tell you straight to your face. He was brutally honest. He was always at the pub, loved a beer – he was your typical old-school hard b*stard.

Although he was well into his seventies and suffering from poor health, his mind was still sharp and we got on well because we could talk about farming, and I appreciated his direct style. Over the years he was always curious about how my farming was going, and he had a great deal of empathy during the tough times. The conversations usually turned towards how and why some things in life and farming had changed, and how others had remained more or less the same. We were on the same wavelength, and we shared a mutual respect.

On his 50th wedding anniversary, there was a celebration at the pub with all of his family there. Out came the cake and he began to talk. As he talked about how much he loved his family, he became very emotional – it was the first time I had ever seen an older man crying, quite openly.

I was shocked and surprised because it was the opposite of the man I had come to know. But more than that, I was blown away by his courage and strength to be so open with his emotions. I had not cried in years, and yet here was this old fella, with a very tough reputation, being willing to cry and talk about his feelings in front of a crowd of 50 people.

I recall when my paternal grandfather died, my father was visibly upset, but I don't remember ever seeing him cry, or talk about it much. It was not how it worked back then.

My takeaway from seeing Nicole's grandfather cry was that he was strong enough to show his vulnerability. I'd had moments in my life since being a kid where I'd felt the overwhelming urge to cry, but felt I couldn't – even on my own – let it out. There was always this feeling, deep down, that would force me to keep my emotions in, no matter how much they needed to come out. The moment I saw Kev crying in front of his family, and saying whatever he felt like saying, was an eye-opener. I'd considered us cut from the same cloth – stoic, tough, old school – so it forced me to ask myself: 'If he can, why can't I?'

I've got huge respect for men who can show their emotions, and that night I saw it demonstrated by someone I deeply respected, and I recognised the strength it took.

It made me connect Kev's emotions with an age-old problem faced by men, particularly rural men: the failure to ask for help.

There are many types of vulnerability but, at that stage in life, I don't think I displayed many of them at all. That day got me thinking about the problem of men not talking. Most guys like me hadn't seen it demonstrated by their male role models. Why couldn't I be the person to overcome that limitation within myself, and model it for others?

There are approximately two million men in New Zealand. Ask yourself: are you going to be the average, or the exception? The exception is the 10 to 15 per cent of men who, by my reckoning, would consider themselves strong enough to be vulnerable. The other 85 per cent live on their pride and let that restrict them.

I don't want to be average – I want to be in the top tier. That's been the way I've approached everything I've done, from farming, to fitness, or just my life; average isn't for me. So I've got to accept that my pride can hold me back. There's much more strength in vulnerability. It's like a little superpower.

Getting in a farm consultant or asking a neighbour for advice are both examples of showing vulnerability.

I think back to my early days in farming, or my rugby playing days, and wish I'd asked more questions. I played rugby with guys who had played provincial rugby for Taranaki, or Super 12 for the Hurricanes, but I never asked them how to train, or advice for positioning on the field. I was too proud, too worried that I would ask something stupid, or be dismissed. I think back now and realise how stupid that was.

When I began dairy farming, there were some very experienced and capable farmers around me but, again, I struggled to ask them questions because I didn't want to look stupid. I tell young farmers now that the only dumb question is the one you don't ask. I could have learned so much from those people, but I didn't.

I wasn't prepared to take the risk because I was uncertain what others would think of me, and I didn't want to face the possibility of a negative answer. These worries were amplified when it came to my emotions, because they are the most powerful and vulnerable feelings.

At Fieldays last year a young guy randomly messaged me on Instagram, asking if I could give him a ride to the event.

I was staying at my brother's farm just out of Rotorua, which meant an early start and a long drive to beat the traffic jam to get in once the gates opened. It was a little out of my way to pick him up and drop him off, but I told him I would meet him at 5.30am in Rotorua. I figured that would be too early for him but, to my surprise, he was there waiting for me, full of enthusiasm. 'Here's a good keen man,' I said to myself.

I gave him a ride simply because he dared to ask. He had the time of his life, meeting all the people he followed on Instagram, and four of us took him out for dinner. I think he had a cool day. I thought: 'Good on you for asking, mate' –

because never in a million years would I have done the same thing at his age. He asked questions all day and got a lot out of the experience. While that may not look like vulnerability to some, he had the courage to ask a virtual stranger for help. While he was with me he displayed courage, and that was the first – and biggest – hurdle to get over when trying to show vulnerability.

The second part of showing vulnerability, or using that courage, is to understand the risk factor, and get over it. There's always a risk people may laugh at you, judge you, act differently towards you, or have a negative reaction when you display vulnerability.

But the reality is that most people are too worried about themselves and what they have going on internally to really give much of a sh*t about you. We worry too much about how others react to us. If they react negatively, so what? They are probably trying to distract from their own problems and failures – like school bullies in the playground. I became aware of this characteristic in people and now, when I weigh up the risks to show my vulnerability, I can still see that the rewards outweigh any risks. In fact, the negative consequences on me of not showing vulnerability have been a pretty heavy burden to carry for most of my life.

Uncertainty is the final hurdle to being vulnerable. It goes hand-in-hand with risk. That's life. Every option, decision, or turn we take in life has risks and rewards – and they all carry uncertainty. We have to understand and get comfortable with being uncertain – accept it is a non-negotiable part of life – and that trying to avoid it means we miss out on more rewards. But the risk will still remain somewhere.

As I became aware of how I backed away from situations requiring vulnerability, I tried to be mindful of the barriers that arose during those moments and I tried to have the courage to take small steps, so it didn't become overwhelming. I began learning by asking simple questions, taking the risk of answering a question with a feeling and, over time, I've become much more comfortable. It's still hard to do ... but, as always in life, the things we know we should do aren't easy.

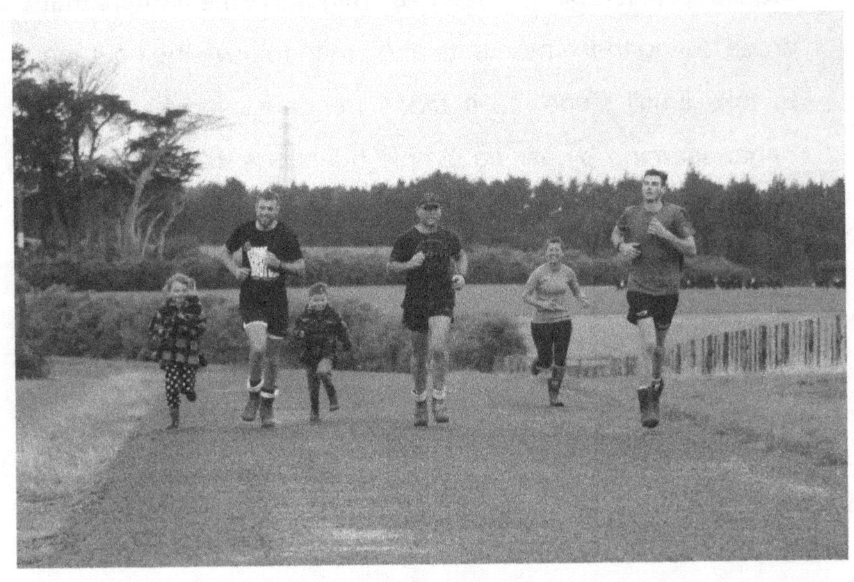

*The Slog Jog for Hope. Left to right: Ahli, me, Parker, Glen Wingate, Nicola Carver, Quintin Adlam.*
(Photo by Maree Saxton)

# Acknowledgements

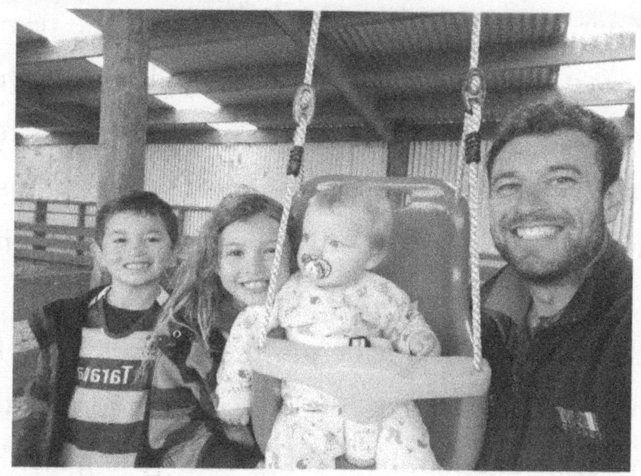

*Me and the kids getting the calf sheds ready for the new season*

There are so many people that have given me something that make up the fibres that are me and my story. Whether it's through a simple conversation, a shared meal or yarns over a beer – I've taken something from you, and this is my way of passing it on. A special thank you to the rural communities of Whenuakura and Ohangai – it's the people who make it so special.

Mum and Dad, for your unwavering support and absolute honesty, it has meant the world to me, and I couldn't have asked for better parents. Nathan and Miah, you've both been great role models and influential in who I am, often showing me what not to do, but being there when it counts. My best mates Andrew, Taylor, Chris, Jayden and Nick for providing laughs when I needed it the most.

Tangaroa Walker, for your words, inspiration and advice. Laura Koot, for your feedback and advice. The team at NZ Farming for everything you do, and to all who have shared stories or messaged me when a part of my story has resonated with you. It's another log on the fire. HarperCollins for the opportunity I had never even dreamed about, and Steve Kilgallon for turning my rambles into a book.

Uncle Ian and Nana McCaul, there was nobody better to show me the Kiwi farming lifestyle, and I'm forever thankful. Martyn Dickie and family, thank you for giving me the start I needed. Brian Williams and family, I'll be forever grateful for the opportunity you provided for me and my family.

Nicole, what a hell of a journey we've had. Thank you for being you – there's no one else that could have done it with me, and I wouldn't have it any other way. Lastly, my children – Ahli, Parker and Dempsey – you always have, and always will be my shining light in the dark, my reason.

**Steve Kilgallon would like to thank:** Alex Hedley for commissioning this book, and, as always, my family, Henry, Alistair, Rosa and Emma.